WEAR
Your Life
WELL

ALSO BY MARILU HENNER

Marilu Henner's Total Health Makeover

The 30-Day Total Health Makeover

I Refuse to Raise a Brat

Healthy Life Kitchen

Healthy Kids

Party Hearty

By All Means Keep on Moving

WEAR
Your Life
WELL

USE WHAT YOU HAVE
TO GET WHAT YOU WANT

MARILU HENNER

WITH LORIN HENNER

Collins

An Imprint of HarperCollins*Publishers*

All efforts have been made to ensure the accuracy of the information contained in this book as of the date published. The author and the publisher expressly disclaim responsibility for any adverse effects arising from the use or application of the information contained herein.

Designed by Kris Tobiassen

ISBN-13: 978-0-06-039365-6
ISBN-10: 0-06-039365-3

For Michael, Nick, and Joey
The best reasons for wearing my life well

Contents

INTRODUCTION xi

The Fifteen Keys to Living Your Life Well

One

**GETTING OUT OF YOUR COMFORT ZONE:
THE FUN OF FACING YOUR FEARS!** 1

My Comfort Zone • Embracing Your Fears • "Face Your Fears" Questionnaire:
What Are You Afraid Of? • Fear of Losing Weight • Fear of Success • Fear of
Change • Fear of Not Being Perfect • Fear of Death/Illness/Information • Fear
of Failure • Forgiving Yourself • Therapy • Wrapping It Up!

Two

**NAVIGATING THE "MINDFIELDS"
OF SELF-SABOTAGE**...25

Emotional Eating • Food Is Seductive • Misplaced Anger • The Power of Body
Armor • Avoiding Sexuality • Jealousy • Self-Sabotage and PMS • What Can I

Get Away With? • Fear of Success (That Ugly Fear Again!) • Self-Sabotage and Control • Lack of Imagination • B-L-A-S-T: Bored, Lonely, Angry, Starving, or Tired • How to Resolve Self-Sabotage • Wrapping It Up!

Three

LEARN TO LOVE THE FOOD THAT LOVES YOU—DETOX 101 49

Change Your Palate, Change Your Life! • Getting Rid of the Health Robbers • Wet Foods versus Concentrated Foods • Centered Foods • The Effects of a Night of Heavy Drinking • Helping Your Doctor Help You • The Best Prescription for Your Own Hands-On Health • The Danger of "Normal" • Time Can Be on Your Side • Wrapping It Up!

Four

SETTING UP YOUR ENVIRONMENT TO *WIN* 83

If You Build It, You Will Become • Your Morning Routine • Snooze Alarm • Morning People • Setting Up Your Kitchen—To Win! • Setting Up Your Bathroom—To Win! • Setting Up Your Closet—To Win! • Setting Up Your Bedroom—To Win! • Setting Up Your Garage—To Win! • Setting Up Your Transportation—To Win! • Wrapping It Up!

Five

THE ROLE OF YOUR LIFE 103

Acting Healthy • Exercise 1: Finding Self with Self • Exercise 2: Observation • Exercise 3: Food for Thought • Exercise 4: The Rant • Exercise 5: Sense Memory • Exercise 6: Character Development • Exercise 7: Finding Your Objective • Exercise 8: Props and Costumes • Exercise 9: Light of Day • Wrapping It Up!

Six

RADAR, RESILIENCE, PLAN B, AND TEFLON 135

The Art of Listening • Positive Breeds Positive, Negative Breeds Negative • Embracing Plan B • Resilience and Teflon • Wrapping It Up!

Seven

USE IT OR LOSE IT 151

Use Your Brain! • Use Your Body • My Exercise Routine • Taking Action • Wrapping It Up!

Eight

SHARPEN YOUR PRESENTATION 163

Communication Skills • Expert Advice • It's All about Homework • Detox Your Style • Wrapping It Up!

Nine

FALL IN LOVE WITH YOUR STRESS—OR IT WILL KILL YOU!   179

Choosing a Familiar…Misery • Don't Be a Lemming • Wrapping It Up!

Ten

THE SEXIEST ORGAN IS . . . YOUR BRAIN! 193

Thinking Sexy • The Pleasure Principle • Wrapping It Up!

Eleven

THE BOOTY CAMP BLITZ 203

Booty Camp Blitz 5-Day Contract • Booty Camp Blitz—Gimme 5! 5-Day Menu • Booty Camp Menu • Booty Camp Recipes

APPENDIX: MARILU HENNER'S FOOD-COMBINING CHARTS 249

ACKNOWLEDGMENTS 253

INDEX 257

Introduction

Years ago I was having lunch with my good friend Jim Brooks, the brilliant three-time Oscar and nineteen-time Emmy Award–winning director and writer. We get together a few times a year, ever since our old *Taxi* days, and he is one of my favorite people, not only because he is brilliant and funny, but also because he is genuinely interested in everything, *especially* the inner workings of the human mind. (You gotta love a guy like that!) So here we were sitting and having a great old time when we both happened to notice a woman a few tables away. She was beautiful, fit, and well dressed and could have been a model from a magazine article on "having it all." Except for one thing.

Everything about her mood said, "I hate my life."

I'm sure she was just having a bad day (and certainly I've had my share of days when I could've looked the same to nosy restaurant patrons), but the sight of her gave the two of us plenty of food for thought and discussion. "Why do you think she's unhappy?" Jim asked, ever the inquisitor. "I have no idea, but it looks like life is wearing her down. Her life is wearing her, rather than the other way around. We've all been there. But it's not enough just to wear your life; you have to wear your life well!"

Jim and I talked a lot that day about what "wear your life well" means, and over the years I've thought about that phrase many times, especially when I see someone worn down by life or feel that way myself. What I've come to realize is that the key to wearing your life well is to fully understand *what you have* and, equally important, know *what you want*. You have to take a profound look at your dreams, goals, and aspirations, followed by a good, hard look at your assets, resources, liabilities, and talents. And then, you have to figure out a way to bridge *the gap between the two*—while learning to enjoy the adventure!

We all know people who seem to have it all—great job, home, family, and so on—but every time you talk to them, they sound miserable. A lot of this negativity radiates from how someone was raised and what he or she was taught to expect from life. Those who grew up thinking the world owes them something, or that life should not be a struggle, tend to struggle their whole lives. On the other hand, there are many people who don't seem to have very much, or are loaded down with many responsibilities, but it doesn't matter. They love life! Every time you see them, they're smiling. They're always optimistic, and they have great faith in their resources and relationships. They can see the bigger picture, and it looks damn good. Struggling doesn't matter to them, because they are wearing their life well. They know how to make things work for them, and you get the feeling that they wouldn't change places with anyone else, because they genuinely love what life has to offer!

The question "How much do you love your life?" is perhaps the best indicator of how well you are wearing yours.

Are you happy? Are you living the life you want? If not, for whom are you doing it all? Are you living for other people? Are you guided by your own plan or by the design of others? Do you see your life as a daily grind, or are you eager to face each day and every new challenge? Do you get along well with your family, friends, relatives, and coworkers, or do you harbor anger, resentment, or guilt? Are you working toward a dream, or are you daydreaming about *not* working? Are you "working the coat," or burying yourself within it? In essence, do you *wear your life well*?

If you are wearing your life as if it came off the rack, how much are you willing to change that? You have to honestly ask yourself *what is and isn't working*. You have to analyze your life from every angle and be willing to make some hard choices, even if it means shaking up someone else's life in the process. Chances are, whatever is *not* working for you is not working for them either, but neither of you has been willing to risk the change. You can't be afraid to be honest with yourself and others. This book may force you to be more truthful than ever before, but I promise it will be worth it!

For the last ten years, I have been creating and teaching weekly classes on diet, fitness, career, and lifestyle on my Web site, Marilu .com. These are very intensive, highly supportive discussions and workshops that have led to an abundance of life-changing moments for me and for thousands of members around the world. Believe me, in ten years, we have talked about *everything*, but the variety of topics we've explored together could be categorized into several basic themes. The more deeply we explored these subjects, the more I realized that mastering all of them is fundamental for living life to the fullest and wearing your life well. I've used these classes to prepare the chapters of this book, so that I can include the wealth of information I have gained over the years from our members. These issues, and the classes that cover them, are the backbone of this book.

The classes at Marilu.com change frequently throughout the year, and there are some classes the members can't get enough of, especially the ones we explore in depth in this book: "The Mindfields of Self Sabotage"; "Getting Out of Your Comfort Zone and Facing Your Fears"; "Learn to Love the Food That Loves You"; "Detox 101"; "Setting Up Your Environment to *Win*"; "The Role of Your Life— YOU, the Character You Were Meant to Play"; "Radar and Resilience; Use It or Lose It"; "Loving Your Stress Before It Kills You"; "Sharpen Your Presentation and Detox Your Style"; "Booty Camp Blitz" (for when you need to get in shape *fast!*); and our favorite subject . . . "SEX"!

Not long after I started working on this book, doing research and interviews and gathering and organizing material, I was offered the opportunity to be on the show *Celebrity Apprentice*. I was concerned at first about putting the book on hold, but then I realized that working on two projects at the same time often benefits both rather than hindering either. I realized, too, that almost every book I've written was crafted while working on another project. I wrote *Total Health Makeover* while starring in the show *Chicago* on Broadway. I was doing *Chicago* again, this time in Las Vegas, while writing *I Refuse to Raise a Brat*. *Healthy Life Kitchen* was written while I was shooting a TV movie. I did the national tour of *Annie Get Your Gun* while writing *Healthy Kids*, and I was working on Broadway in *The Tale of the Allergist's Wife* while writing *Healthy Holidays*. This book turned out to be no exception.

I'm glad I took on *Celebrity Apprentice* in the middle of writing this book, because it gave me a perspective I would not have had otherwise. Sometimes in life you're set on a path, and you don't even know why you're following, it but you trust the world and your instincts enough to know that the reason will eventually reveal itself. It turned out that I could not have had a more perfect experience to correlate with this book. I learned more about myself and others by observing how we all handled being tested in such a cutthroat, stressful, time-condensed environment. It was more than gratifying to me to realize that everything I was writing about rang true with the celebrities I was competing against. It was a powerful reconfirmation of the core philosophies of this book, because I watched them all in *action*!

Every person on the show was dealing with comfort zones, self-sabotage, and facing their fears. Many people showed how well they use what they have to get what they want. I witnessed those who were quick-witted and dynamic at tasks because they trusted themselves to stay "in the moment." I could see evidence that the most successful people were those who had learned how to use it, not lose it. I recognized the advantage of knowing how to set up your environment to win. I saw time and time again that presentation was even more important than what was being presented. I watched people who were brilliant at tuning into their radar, and those who failed themselves and others because they didn't know how to read a room. I witnessed people use their sex appeal to get what they needed in the most attractive ways. I watched people lie, cheat, beg, borrow, and steal—but we were playing a game, and it was all in the name of charity! And I learned again what I've always known: Resilience and being able to "get over it" are the most important qualities to possess in order to get where you most want to go.

But most of all, I learned that, like it or not, you are in charge of your own life. (You're the Project Manager!) If you find that something's not working, it's up to you to make the necessary adjustments. You can assign the other people in your life the necessary tasks to get the job done, but you, and only you, are responsible for making it all work.

The Fifteen Keys to Living Your Life Well

Ever since my lunch with Jim Brooks, I've been making a list of what it takes to wear your life well. I've added to the list as I've taught the classes at Marilu.com and have seen what works for others—as well as what I've learned the hard way myself! Chapter by chapter we'll be exploring the ones I feel are the most imperative for helping you use what you have to get what you want.

You have to:

1. Identify, "de-trigger," and get over the self-sabotage.
2. Get along with the important people in your life.
3. Learn to love the food that loves you.
4. Set up your environment to win.
5. Know the basic elements of detox.
6. Figure out if you're a thinker, a speaker, or a writer. And then you have to do it every day to ask for what you want.
7. Find "the juice," the excitement, in what you do.
8. Be able to coat yourself in Teflon when dealing with other people.
9. Learn to access your brain cells so that you are in present time.
10. Go for the *light* instead of the *dark* in any given situation.
11. Stay on top of things—your health, your home, your work, your looks, and your people.
12. Fall in love with your stress, or it will kill you.
13. Preserve your resources so that you can keep doing the things you love to do for a long time.
14. Get in sync with the sexual you.
15. Have a five-day blitz in your back pocket when you want to get in shape fast!

You are at the beginning of a great journey. Expect many challenges, detours, and key insights along the way. You will undoubtedly discover things about yourself and the people close to you that will profoundly change your perspective and direction. Isn't it time to use what you have to get what you want and start wearing your life well?

WEAR

Your Life

WELL

One

GETTING OUT OF YOUR COMFORT ZONE: THE FUN OF FACING YOUR FEARS!

What do you *truly* want to do with your life? Have you ever *really* figured it out? I'm not just asking what you want to be when you grow up. This has more to do with your overall life design and covers more territory than just your career. This includes everything—your family, education, diet, health, free time, hobbies, friends, home, travel, even your mission statement. I mean, in theory we all know what we want in our lives, and most people are deeply rooted in the lifestyle they're already living—whether or not they're happy about that! But have you ever truly thought this through and conceived in detail your ideal life, without thinking about the obstacles to or consequences of actually pulling it off? Doing this could become the most important exercise you've ever undertaken.

If you really could design your ideal life, how close would it be to the life you're living right now? When asked this question, most people propose a life with *more* than they now have, which usually means a bigger and better house, a more successful and rewarding career, more time to spend with family, more money, owning a business, being famous—the list is endless. We naturally want more, but we rarely factor in the *consequences* of having more. There are responsibilities that automatically come with having more in your life, and even though we don't always consciously think about it, we are aware of it *sub*consciously. Deep down we know that these responsibilities challenge what we've already set up in our cozy little comfort zones.

The risk of losing some of our comfort in life plays a prominent role in our efforts to attain our goals. We know that changing our lives for the better may come with a price tag, and that price is more responsibility, leading to more stress, and therefore *less* comfort. It's difficult to create the life you want until you identify, control, or at least understand your own comfort zones. You also need to be aware of your life goals, so you can recognize which comfort zones you're protecting—and which responsibilities or burdens you may be avoiding.

My Comfort Zone

Everyone has his or her own unique comfort zones that come in all shapes and sizes. I have some that are significant and others that are trivial. My silliest comfort zone is the way I like to sleep. For years people have teased me about my sleeping requirements—a room so dark you never know what time it is. (Elvis would have been proud!) In fact, I have "blackout shades requested" written into every location contract I sign, but not because I'm a diva. I need to sleep in a dark room because I *love* to be awake! Any hint of light represents action, and I automatically want to be part of that action. If there's so much as a firefly out there, I'm ready to party!

No matter how crazy my sleeping comfort zone seems to others, it's certainly better than my eating comfort zone was years ago, before I got healthy and lost fifty-five pounds. Back then I lived under the tyranny of stupid diets, thinking that alternating deprivation with gluttony was the way to go. The discomfort of being heavy and bloated all the time was even part of this comfort zone. It was only after I acquired the necessary knowledge and retrained my palate that my eating comfort zone changed.

In figuring out how to use what you have to get what you want, it's necessary to take an honest look at your whole life and see where you're at, right here, right now.

What are *your* comfort zones? What have you set up in your life to support the good and bad behaviors that make you "you"? How do you relate to everyone and everything around you, from your eating patterns to your sleeping rituals, your exercise routines to your clothing choices, your relationship strategies to the way you think and feel about yourself? What are *your* habits that may even feel comfortably uncomfortable? What made you set up certain conditions so that you can continue to succeed . . . or fail? And where did you learn *how* to set up these conditions? Are you mimicking your parents? Rebelling against your family? Or have you just learned the best way to survive?

Looking at other people's lives, you may often think, *I could never live like that. Their schedule is too crazy. Their house is too chaotic. Their relationship is too dramatic.* Yet, when you look closely, you see that it works for them! We all have those quirky things we think we need in our lives in order to survive. If someone took away your comfort zone, what would be your backup? Would you need one? Or would it be better if you were forced to give it up with nothing to replace it?

You get interesting answers when you ask people, "What does the phrase 'comfort zone' mean to you?" The responses will vary, but what is most telling is that each person mentions first the area of his or her life that needs the most help. Many people talk about their relationships, and yet pick the same unhappy situation over and over again. It proves that we all know what we're trying to get away with, and that we're not fooling anyone—least of all ourselves!

The point is to challenge yourself to get *out* of your comfort zones if staying in one doesn't move your life forward. Staying in your comfort zone seems to be one of the main barriers to achieving your goals, because it keeps you rigid and less adaptable to diversity and change. When you're in a comfort zone, you'll tend to do the same things over and over because it's easy. You know what to expect and how to respond without thinking.

But what if you really like everything just the way it is? Is there anything wrong with staying in your comfort zone to keep it that way? Well, possibly not. But does anyone *really* want to keep everything in his or her world exactly the way it is? Do you really want the same old boring path of least resistance? That can become dull awfully fast, and eventually you lose sight of all the possibilities you're missing out on because you're no longer exposed to better alternatives, including healthier, more varied, sometimes simpler, and sometimes more innovative choices. Protecting your comfort zone also tends to support bad habits rather than helping you find new ways to navigate your life by allowing healthier habits to become a part of it.

I think many people are afraid to challenge their comfort zones because they know, consciously or subconsciously, that change caused them a certain amount of stress in the past. Even though we usually gain something from taking these risks, we are reluctant to test those boundaries again because of the uncertainty and stress we associate with the unknown. The sad part is that this becomes more of a problem as we get older. Kids don't have nearly as much stress over leaving their comfort zones as adults do. They are much more adventurous because they haven't quite settled into their comfort zones yet. People over sixty have an especially difficult time leaving their CZs. (Try talking your grandmother into changing the meat-based diet she's been eating all her life!)

So, here's what I suggest. Don't think of challenging your comfort zones as something that you have to force yourself to do. With that attitude, you'll end up avoiding change altogether. Instead, think of each new challenge or change as an exciting new adventure. Try to recapture the innocent, non-jaded enthusiasm you had as a child. Don't overanalyze and worry about failing or having a bad experience. Whatever your new endeavor is, take it all in as part of the experience. Think of every comfort zone detour as a mini-vacation from yourself, and don't get upset if the hypothetical "hotel room" outside your comfort zone is noisy or doesn't face the pool!

Testing these boundaries can actually be a lot of fun! And remember, there are many subcategories to your comfort zone—your health, love life, family, finances, career, and so on. Each has its own defined comfort zone. Here are just a few suggestions to help get you started:

- In the food category, try a vegetable you've never tried before. If you're always making the same old side dish, like steamed broccoli, try preparing something totally new, such as daikon or jicama. Ask for advice from your produce manager, or do a little research on the Internet about choosing and preparing a new, exotic vegetable. We often avoid trying a new vegetable because we don't know how to wash, cut, or prepare it. That's out of our comfort zone. Don't just limit this change to a new vegetable. Try new kinds of fruit, grains, beans, and pasta. And don't just fix the same old pasta sauce; ask your friends to share some of their favorites. Prepare a new recipe every week. We stay with our old standbys because it's easier; we know exactly what to buy and how to prepare it. To spice things up a bit, try a recipe from another country or culture. Your family might just love the surprise. Don't be afraid to botch it up. That might even add to the fun.

- In the discipline department, try having a sugar-free, dairy-free, meat-free, or fast food–free day (or entire week or month if you're more advanced). This is a great way to explore how much better you would feel if you ate a cleaner diet.

- In the lifestyle category, consider reading a book in a subject you know nothing about. We tend to explore areas we're already familiar with because it's easier; it's in our comfort zone. Try a weekend getaway that's very different, too. Surprise your spouse—don't give him or her a chance to nix the new choice; everyone needs their comfort zones pushed! And make sure you keep an open mind throughout the experience.

- When it comes to exercise, I'm a firm believer in lots of variety. Fitness gains are much greater when your body is challenged with variation in resistance and movement. Physical improvements come from changeups in your routine. So explore new sports, dance classes, and exercises you've never done before. Do remember, however, to be cautious if you're doing anything a bit risky, unless you *want* to end up in traction, which, by the way, is the ultimate comfort zone!

Being part of *Celebrity Apprentice* was a lesson in observing others and their comfort zones. Celebrities are known for negotiating into their contracts the little, and not so little, requests that make it easier to do their jobs. Often these requests are so over-the-top they are legendary. (Remember Michael Jackson's alleged oxygen chamber required for his dressing room, or Marilyn Manson's kitty litter box in lieu of the . . . well . . . loo?) Before we even started filming, a celebrity liaison called and asked our requirements in terms of food, drink, other amenities, and so on. I'm always very careful about my food, so I, of course, requested that we would be able to get healthy meals while on the go. I knew that we'd be working long and strenuous hours, and I wanted to make sure that I could eat the healthy food that I know is easily available in New York.

On the very first day, we were asked to submit a list of the foods we wanted in our War Rooms, the rooms where each team would be spending most of its time brainstorming. The list was as diverse as the people. One part of the group asked for every sweet, cheesy, meaty, unhealthy food and snack they could get their hands on—the junkier the better. And two of us on the team could not have been more opposite in our requests, including asking for fresh organic vegetables and a juicer!

I was amazed that some people could wolf down cheeseburgers, french fries, candy, cheese things, and banana splits—in the ten minutes they gave us to eat—and still try to think clearly. Temperature was another biggie. The War Rooms were on the same floor, and although we couldn't hear each other, we were connected by a heating and air-conditioning system. Our team was always freezing and wanted to blast the heat, so of course, we'd constantly get a knock on the door from Vinnie Pastore or one of the producers saying, "It's too hot in the guys' room! What's with all the heat in there, girls?" The guys with all their muscle and mass were always hot, and the women with their smaller frames and lighter clothing were always cold.

The battles between the sexes were not just about managing, marketing, and selling; it came down to a basic difference in day-to-day survival. We would occasionally share each other's rooms for group or board meetings, and the contrast between the two rooms was obvious. The women's room was always immaculate and organized, and the guys' room was disheveled and filthy. Whenever I was in their War Room, I was too creeped out to even use their restroom. There was always a little bit of pee on the toilet seat and on the floor surrounding the toilet. Tissues piled up without being thrown out, and none of the guys seemed to mind . . . or even notice! The guys' CZ was so different from the girls'. You can be sure that Mars is a lot dirtier than Venus. It turns out that the sulfuric fumes we have detected from Mars are *not* from volcanoes! We also could not have been more diverse in terms of the way we approached being project manager and getting the best or worst out of our teammates. Some people were able to adjust to whatever the conditions were, while others had to have a certain state of chaos in order to succeed. This is not unusual. I've worked with actors in the past who were notorious for creating an on-set atmosphere that was tumultuous for everyone, but because of the turmoil and tension, they were able to shine at everyone else's expense.

The TV show *Project Runway* is also a lesson in observing other people's comfort zones. Other reality shows use a similar strategy, but on *Project Runway*, it's not only a question of outwitting, outlasting, and outplaying; you also have to create something that is special and beautiful and wears well—every week! Imagine what it would be like to be uprooted from your home, live with strangers, compete with your roommates for lots of money and a big opportunity, and still have to marshal your creative energies to design something special and beautiful that wears well—like your *health*!

As you read this book, keep in mind that your goal should be not only to push the envelope of your usual routine but also to learn to protect what you need to succeed.

Embracing Your Fears

What scares you? What are you afraid of? What wakes you up in the middle of the night, grabs your imagination, and keeps you from falling back to sleep as you play out various scenarios to their illogical conclusions? When I'm afraid of something, the writer in me loves to imagine every twist and turn my fear can drive me through; the actress in me puts myself in every role my fear will allow me to play.

Sometimes we fear what we feel we aren't good at, can't commit to, or are reluctant to learn. We're afraid to look awkward, silly, or uncoordinated, so we play it safe and do nothing. There are always going to be fears; you'll always be afraid of something. It's just a matter of what kind of emotional muscle you're willing to develop in order to be able to handle those fears and then move on with your life. If you can turn your fear around and learn to use what you're afraid of, then your fear can often propel you to make a huge difference in your life. You'll then be able to change your perception enough to open up and present yourself in a way that may not necessarily make you comfortable but at least won't let you hide forever.

Let's say, for example, that you're reluctant to go to the gym because you're afraid everyone is looking at you. Suppose you mentally prepared yourself for that fear by imagining yourself in that situation and then decided how you were going to handle it? What if you went to the gym and pretended that no one else mattered? You could say to yourself, "I know there are going to be people looking at me, but I'm going to look my fellow gym members in the eye and smile. I'm going to work out even harder than usual and enjoy the fact that I'm on display. I'm going to be excited to be what everyone else is thinking about today!"

It's unlikely that you'll ever see half the people in the gym again, so even if people are looking (and don't think for a second they aren't, because you're doing it, too), what's the big deal? We all look, compare, judge, and then think, "Oh, I'm not as bad as he or she is." After that, most people go home and eat ice cream to celebrate their superiority. The next time you're self-conscious at the gym, think of all the people going home to eat ice cream after seeing you and how, in a month, you're going to be the fit one! Look at it this way: Fear on your face isn't going to make you look any more attractive, but confidence and gusto will! A great attitude is contagious, but if there's no one at the gym who wants to jump on the Gusto bandwagon, then let them be reminded of their own self-consciousness when they see a confident you! People's first reaction to seeing someone who is self-assured is usually, "Wow! That person's got something!"

Have you ever looked at an old class photo from grade school, and when you've shown people your classmates, they pick out someone and say, "This is a pretty girl," or "That boy was cute"? And you tell them, "What? That kid? No way! She was kind of picked on," or "She was mean," or "He was a nerd." Then you realize that your image of them has to do not with how they looked, but with how they behaved. This scenario is just as true for adults. We think the way we look matters more than our attitude, but it's the exact opposite. Now, that's not to say that we shouldn't be our best, or try to look good and be healthy. This isn't a license to be a "nice" bad eater. But while you're learning the tools that will make you more balanced, healthier, more fit, and better looking, it doesn't mean you can't improve your attitude to help speed up the process.

I used to be afraid that if I weren't hard on myself, I would quickly fall apart. As a result, I fell in love with being hard on myself. Being "your own worst critic" doesn't have to be a bad thing, because you then only have to worry about judging yourself. Why be concerned about anyone else's harsh opinion if you're the tough one? If done properly, being your own worst (best!) critic can bring about great success. You'll be setting your own bar high enough to consistently improve your personal best. But don't be afraid to be good to yourself, either. It isn't the same as giving up, unless being "good" means allowing indulgent behaviors that are actually self-destructive.

It's best to have a glass-half-full attitude about everything you do. Lighten up and learn to laugh at yourself. It's amazing how many of your fears go away when you have a sense of humor about them. I've learned as an actress that there are two things you lose when you're scared—your humor and your sexuality. They go right out the window! Fear really starts in your head, and if you really want to overcome your fears, you first have to turn them around in that powerful brain of yours first.

As you read this book, you'll be confronted with the same types of questions I've asked myself over the years in order to dig deep enough to change my life. Self-examination is never easy, but when you read or hear something that reroutes your thinking and inspires you to move in a more positive direction, then every step of the journey becomes more gratifying than the next.

"Face Your Fears" Questionnaire: What Are You Afraid Of?

1. Are you afraid to look in the mirror?
2. Are you afraid your "fat" clothes are becoming your wardrobe?
3. Are you afraid that you're getting too comfortable in your rut?
4. Are you afraid of making your friends jealous?
5. Are you afraid to stand up to your mother-in-law (or someone else) with your new healthy habits?
6. Are you afraid of your own anger?

7. Are you afraid of spending time on yourself?

8. Are you afraid of never being the person you know you can be?

9. Are you afraid to be your best—or that your best won't be good enough?

10. Are you afraid of getting caught "faking it"?

11. Are you afraid of your own limitations?

12. Are you afraid of facing your mistakes without eating your feelings?

13. Are you afraid to say "No!" to your inner brat?

14. Are you afraid of admitting it's time to change?

15. Are you afraid to see a doctor about something you know is wrong?

16. Are you afraid of having too much information?

17. Are you afraid good health will never be yours?

18. Are you afraid of knowing too much about yourself?

19. Are you afraid that the best thing in your life is food?

20. Are you afraid if you give up dieting, you'll have to devote time to your other "talents"?

21. Are you afraid of what "success" would mean to your life?

22. Are you afraid that "getting healthy" won't work for you?

Taking a deep breath and admitting to a list of things that scared me in that first Face Your Fears class is one of the most truly brave things I've ever done, and it was so freeing. Making major changes in your health and your life can bring up all kinds of fears—deprivation, rejection, not belonging—and owning those fears is the first step toward conquering them.

—TONIA
KULBERDA,
New Jersey,
Marilu.com
member

The Face Your Fears classes made me see the things I never really took the time to confront or even notice.

—FAITH WAIT,
Pennsylvania,
Marilu.com
member

Fear of Losing Weight

People often tell me that one of their biggest fears has to do with losing weight. Aside from the physical change, they fear their entire lives would change, and perhaps not in a positive way. People might be jealous, spouses might feel threatened, and their own personality might become arrogant and insensitive. There's also the fear that the pressure would be too much and they couldn't keep up their new routine. It's too much to maintain a healthy lifestyle.

Been there. Done that.

I used to think these very thoughts before figuring out the Total Health Makeover (THM) program. I struggled when I needed to lose weight for a particular purpose, such as a job or an event, and then I'd blow it all out after the period of deprivation was over. I'd appease myself by thinking, "I'm just big!" which was easier than actually changing my eating habits for good. I used every excuse in the book until I realized I was spending year after year stuck in the same spot. When I ran out of excuses, I started doing the work. Most of all, I recognized that my life wasn't some movie with the credits about to roll. Nothing was static. I was an ever-evolving creature, and I could change and grow and inspire jealousy, and be arrogant one minute and empathetic the next. I was alive! And my weight problem was really mine and in my head and on my body, and no one was paying as much attention to it as I was.

Let me ask you this: If you finally got down to the weight you've always wanted to be, what's the first thing you would do? Would you get a different job? Tell someone off? Look up an old flame? Finally take that class you've always wanted to take? Seriously, what would you do differently than you are doing now? What does being the "best you" look like? (And I don't mean just physically.)

Fear of Success

When trying to analyze one's fears, I think the question really is: How authentic do you want to be? How connected do you want to be to the person you really are deep down? Or is that deep down person just an imaginary friend rather than a living, breathing human being?

Which brings us to the fear of success.

Let's say you get into the best shape of your life, and you feel like you can do anything, and your life is finally coming together the way you've always imagined it would.

Then what? What happens next? What does that success look like? And if you fear it, why does it scare you?

Or do you say, "Bring it on!"?

I used to deal with my fears by pretending they didn't exist. That took me a long way in doing brave things, but inside I felt like an imposter.

—LYRICAL,
Marilu.com
member

Fear of Change

Let's pretend for a moment that from this day forward, the weight you are *right now* is the weight you will be for the rest of your life.

Think about it.

You would be in the same physical state you are today, no matter how well you ate or how much you worked out. This would be it. You would get older, but you wouldn't get smaller or bigger.

Would you be depressed because you couldn't do anything about it? Or would you be *relieved* because you couldn't do anything about it? After all, there would be no more struggling, no more pressure to change. You would just be the physical you that you are today . . . forever.

Would you live the rest of your life hiding behind the clothes you've recently been wearing? Or would you feel inspired to force yourself into a new style? Would you get that new haircut you've been promising yourself as soon as you lost weight? Would you learn to rock this look? Would you accept yourself as you are today and make the best of it?

What would you do if the ability to change were taken away from you?

Or is *change* still something you fear?

Fear of Not Being Perfect

This fear is a biggie! It's a theme that shows up in various forms during our classes at Marilu.com, and it's one that sneaks insidiously into our psyches and won't let go.

See if you can relate to any of the following statements:

- "I already blew my diet, so I might as well pig out the rest of the day."

- "No matter how much I exercise, I'll never look like ____."

- "My body (house, wardrobe, job) will never be that great, so why try to improve it?"

- "Why bother learning an instrument (or how to cook, or how to paint)? I'll never be that good."

- "I'll never be happy with my life, so why not be depressed?"

That's right. I'm talking about *perfection*! (Or, rather, the fear of not being perfect!) Oh, that word! It can paralyze, suffocate, or destroy you. It can keep you from taking the first step, or trying your best, or even doing anything at all. It's such an issue with people that I made it part of the Total Health Makeover slogan—"Progress, not perfection!" I know how much it can devastate people when they think they're not being "perfect." Perfectionism runs rampant in my family, to the point where an uncle stopped doing *anything* if it couldn't be perfect. His siblings used to say, "Your Uncle Dan is a perfectionist. In other words, he does nothin'!" I'm here to tell you, there is no such thing as perfect. And, as I'm always saying, the only time you're perfect is when you're perfectly dead!

Fear of Death/Illness/Information

Every year during April, my birthday month, I have a routine physical that involves all of the major tests. I love doing this because it tells me exactly what's going on with my body and what I need to adjust from the last year. I've always been the kind of person who loves to know everything. Friends tease me about this, because they know I like all kinds of feedback, good and bad.

But not everyone wants to hear *everything*.

I've seen people so afraid of giving up a vice—whether it's smoking, alcohol, bad food, or an affair—that they refuse to acknowledge commonsense information. I've seen people so afraid of knowing their state of health that they wouldn't see a doctor until it was too late. And I've seen people so afraid of dying that they have kept themselves from living.

How much do you like to know? Is there some vice you know you should give up, but you close your ears to hearing the truth? Are you afraid to see your doctor because he may tell you something you can't handle? And last but not least, does a fear of dying keep you from doing something you would love to do?

Fear of Failure

When I think about the fear of failure, the first thing that comes to mind is something I heard when I was sixteen and I was choreographing a show for a local community theatre. The director's wife was the very talented star of our show, and she had been responsible for my getting the job after seeing me play a small part in one of their earlier productions.

We were backstage one day, and she told me that I reminded her of herself when she was younger (she was probably all of twenty-six at the time). She asked if I was serious about being in show business, going to New York or Hollywood, and I said, "Yes, of course. I see myself in show business, working on Broadway, the whole bit." And I remember that she said to me, "Really? Not me. I don't think I could take it. What if I didn't make it? What if I didn't like it? What if it's not what it should be? Nope. I'm the type who'll be happier thinking how great I *could* have been."

I'll never forget her statement. It seemed so strange to me at the time. I couldn't imagine choosing *imagining* you were great over at least *trying* for greatness.

What about you?

Is it better to at least try, even if you fall short of your mark? Or do you prefer to think how great you *could have* been . . . or looked . . . or felt . . . or succeeded . . . or created something?

Forgiving Yourself

A few years ago I had the good fortune of meeting Kitty Carlisle, the famous actress, opera singer, author, performer, and entrepreneur, who not long ago passed away at the ripe old age of ninety-six. When I met her, she was still performing her club act in New York to sellout crowds. I read an article in which she was asked the secret to her long, successful life. She said that every morning she looks in the mirror, takes a long and hard look at herself, and says, "I forgive you."

When I read that, I stopped dead in my tracks. Those three words can make such a difference in how you spend your day. Do you carry the burden of yesterday's sins? Do you constantly beat yourself up for whatever you did or were the day, week, month, year, decade, before? Or do you look yourself in the eye, say "I forgive you," and move on?

Therapy

Sometimes, most of the time really, you just can't do the major fear-facing alone. I went to therapy for many years starting when I was twenty-three. I figured, "Why wait to be old to be wise?" I was living alone in New York at the time, and I was behaving out of touch and disconnected from my feelings, and I knew I needed some help.

The wrong therapist is worse than no therapist, so it's important to make sure you have a *good* therapist. A general rule of thumb is to find a therapist who respects the contract that you have. For example, if the session is fifty minutes, it shouldn't go over the fifty minutes. A good therapist honors the contract and can help "cure" you by main-taining the rules and boundaries set forth within the contract.

In other words, you don't want to be buddy-buddy with your thera-pist. I had a friend whose sessions with her therapist were often spent doing each other's nails! She called her therapist by her first name, and no session ever took the same amount of time. In fact, most of their "fifty-minute sessions" ran two hours! The therapist was also casual about collecting the fees, and eventually my friend's therapy bill ex-ceeded $6,000, the bulk of which she is still paying. My friend knew she was racking up the charges but figured, "What the heck. I'll pay it off someday." It's not surprising that she still struggles with money and time issues. A therapist can really make a difference in the patient's progress with major life issues by the way he or she respects the contract.

A good therapist is challenging, especially in the beginning, and doesn't give you all the answers. A good therapist encourages you to look deep within yourself to find the answers and helps you put things into proper perspective. In therapy you're there to talk, vent, and dis-cuss. You talk about anything and everything, and, by doing so, you begin to recognize that your feelings are powerful, and by putting your feelings into words you are less likely to put them into action. For example, you can say, "I hate my husband, and I want to kill him!" but by expressing those feelings in therapy, you (hopefully!) don't go out and actually do it. The more you express your feelings, the less likely you are to act on them. A therapist isn't there to judge you, but rather to help you figure it all out. The idea is to be able to express your negative feelings—even about therapy—and still stay in treatment.

I always thought of therapy as being able to go to the greatest com-puter program in the world. You ask it a question, and, in turn, it asks you one, which then requires you to ask yourself more questions, un-til you finally get the answers. The more questions you ask, the more you learn about what's really going on.

Sometimes when you cry, it's really tears of rage. You're upset because you're frustrated at not being able to articulate what you're feeling. I used to get into a session and just cry because I couldn't express myself the way I wanted to. I remember coming out of one of my early sessions, and I was in such a daze from having expressed myself in a way I hadn't before that I walked right into a tree. Therapy definitely stirs things up!

I spent a lot of time working on myself because I knew that I had all this potential living inside me. Once I really got in touch with who I was, and who I wanted to be—and the outside connected with the inside—there was no stopping me! It doesn't happen overnight, though. People think that things are "fixed" in some way, and that once you achieve a goal, it stops there. Getting healthy is an ongoing process. It requires a lot of patience and understanding. It's especially difficult in the beginning when it's hard to see the future healthy you. Later on, when you get to a place where you're starting to feel the results of your labors, you want more of the same, so you keep getting healthier.

I'm writing this not only because I think therapy is worth talking about but also to explain how language can be a very powerful tool against one's fears. You can resolve so much with language. I learned from Dr. Ruth Velikovsky Sharon, coauthor with me of *I Refuse to Raise a Brat,* that your feelings are just your feelings. Your feelings won't kill you. The important thing is to feel all your feelings and then decide which ones to put into action, after you've thought them out well enough to know exactly what you want to do with them. The trick is to *resolve* your feelings rather than just trying to *overcome* them, because otherwise something worse may pop up. For example, someone who is trying to overcome a weight problem may begin to substitute something else—drugs, alcohol, or sex—instead of understanding the underlying causes of the original problem. Years ago, a very overweight friend of mine went on a crazy strict diet that made no sense whatsoever. A few weeks into the diet, when he wasn't happy at all, he developed Bell's palsy and felt he had to get back to his food. It was as if his body rebelled because he hadn't thought through his food obsession and reasons for wanting to overeat in the first place. Eventually he sought counseling, and I was able to help him gradually change some of his eating habits so that he didn't feel overwhelmed. The Bell's palsy never returned, and his health and weight improved.

Ultimately, the goal is to talk about and *understand* your feelings enough so that they don't affect you in a destructive way. You can actually *choose* to carry around the negative baggage, or to work through it using "progress, not perfection" as your mantra, so that it doesn't weigh you down the rest of your life.

Time is a great healer and a great factor in healing.

As you become an adult, you realize that your parents were probably doing the best they could, given where they came from and what they experienced as children. They may also have lived in a time when people didn't have self-help tools available the way we do now. They had fewer privileges than we had, and certainly a lot fewer than our children have. Often, people who have the more difficult upbringings are the most successful, because they know they have to find their own way. As you get older, you realize that you can have the whole roulette wheel of feelings about your parents. It's almost like a "wheel of fortune" that could stop on any characteristic or feeling, and you could think about your parents, or anything for that matter, that way. It's important to know that if you want to be a fully realized human being, you *should* have, *can* have, and *do* have all of your feelings.

I think it's important to try to work out your primary relationships with your family because they are your original "group," and there's so much we take into the rest of the world based on how we related to our family members.

I believe that when certain fears come up, you can talk yourself through them in some way—until you get good at recognizing that the fear is unfounded, irrational, or something that needs to be explored because it's really based on something else. Even though a particular state of being—loneliness, depression, and so on—exists in the foreground, all the other feelings on your "wheel of fortune" are also there and available.

Imagine that you're hanging on a trapeze between two platforms, and you start swinging a little and gaining momentum. Pretty soon, you're swinging more and more between the two extremes. Let's call them, for this example, "staying in the marriage" and "getting a divorce." Those are the names of the platforms, and you're swinging back and forth between the two. In order to finally jump onto one of the platforms, you need to get enough momentum from swinging from the opposite platform. Just when it looks like you'll land on one, you swing all the way over to the other side. You can't land unless you've swung that far in the opposite direction. Sometimes feeling the worst you can about something is the very thing that gives you the momentum to feel the best you can about the same situation. But you have to allow yourself the pain of exploration.

If you are only interested in "feeling better," then that's what makes you numb to life.

People are interested in feeling better because they're so afraid of their negative feelings—about themselves, their spouses, jobs, kids— that all they want is to feel better with something like food. When they are miserable the day after a major pig-out, it's more about the food and the heaviness they suffer than what made them overeat in the first place. Some people's rock bottom can go on forever because they never allow themselves to "feel" rock bottom. Rock bottom doesn't mean having to be a blacked-out alcoholic or dirt poor and living on the streets. Rock bottom could be a person *choosing* to live in front of their television set, never exercising, learning, or growing. A person can hit rock bottom because of their fears.

Have you caught yourself fearing something, and then realized it wasn't so scary after all?

I think we all have this image of the person we *could* be, and when we feel we're not up to the task of being that person, we let our fears hold us back from even trying. When you can work on yourself enough to trust that what you do *can* and *will* make a difference in the world, and you begin to understand that, no matter how down, depressed, lonely, or fat you may feel at any one time, deep in your heart you really know who you are—and it doesn't scare you.

Wrapping It Up!

- It's important to examine what you truly want in your life.

- The risk of losing some of our comfort in life plays a prominent role in our efforts to attain our goals.

- What does the phrase "comfort zone" mean to you?

- What have you set up in your life to support the good and bad behaviors that make you "you"?

- Challenge yourself to get *out* of your comfort zones if staying in one doesn't move your life forward.

- Analyze and make a list of your fears.

- Learn to lighten up and laugh at yourself.

- How authentic do you want to be?

- How would your life change if you reached your goals?

- Don't avoid living because you fear failure.

- Think progress, not perfection.

- Forgive yourself *every* day!

- Getting healthy is an ongoing process. It requires a lot of patience and understanding.

- Talk about and *understand* your feelings enough so that they don't affect you in a destructive way.

Two

NAVIGATING THE "MINDFIELDS" OF SELF-SABOTAGE

One of the first steps to wearing your life well is coming to grips with self-sabotage. You can't move forward on the game board of life if you're constantly stuck on the same space, that nasty little space called self-sabotage! Self-sabotage is insidious because it can manifest itself in any area of your life, including your relationship tactics, career strategies, and food issues. Whatever it is you need to do to improve your life, you can find a novel way to sabotage it.

I've had my share of sabotaging relationships and making dumb decisions in my career, but nothing in my life compares to my old self-sabotaging ways with food! Becoming a healthy, fit person is much easier now than it was when I first started my health journey in the late 1970s. Back then there were no food labels, no nutritious fast foods, and no health food aisles in mainstream grocery stores. Today we have better and more accessible information on everything from alternative medicine to knowing what's inside that can of soup. There really is no excuse for our *not* being as healthy as we can be.

So, what's the problem? Why are we sicker, fatter, and lazier than ever before?

I'll tell you why. Despite all of the great information available to us, we as human beings, with our human frailties, choose to thwart our best efforts, time and time again, with self-sabotage!

But what is self-sabotage, and why does it have such a stranglehold on us?

Self-sabotage is the method we use to set ourselves up to fail. It's the excuse we give when we want to blame our failure on something or someone else. It's the reason we bail on our New Year's resolutions long before January is over, and why we cheat on our diets the moment we start seeing progress. The key to success is in understanding that the urge to self-sabotage can be controlled. We can turn our negative impulses into positive ones, and, once we do, our goals can be achieved.

Self-sabotage is an easy trap to fall into. Before Total Health Make-over, I was so confused by all the conflicting health information out there that I thought I would never have confidence about what I ate. A few weeks into the program, I got it—I really knew what worked, it all made sense, I'd never felt better—but then I immediately thought, "How great that I know what works for me—now I can do this any-time I want." It wasn't until "anytime" became right now—today, this meal, this workout—that I made a real change in my health and fitness.

—CATHY
DODD,
Washington,
Marilu.com
member

Self-sabotage has always been one of my favorite topics because it doesn't matter what stories people have told me; I've already been there. I know what it's like to get within striking distance of my goal weight, only to give up five or ten pounds from the finish line. I know what it's like to pull off a certain look, get compliments, and then give myself permission to blow it. I know what it's like to give in and give up as I get close to what I really want. Self-sabotage lurks within each of us every day of our lives. It has many characteristics, many faces, and many personalities, all with the same objective in mind—to get you off track, away from your goals, and stuffing your face as quickly as possible!

After studying self-sabotage for many years, and finally "curing" myself of this nasty disease, I've come to realize that there are *at least* thirty-three reasons we self-sabotage (see the sidebar), and that we all master at least six of them. Becoming aware of the different reasons is the first step. Paying attention to that initial impulse to get off track is important. Note how many times you feel the urge to go to the refrigerator or pantry throughout the day and you'll start to realize that most of the time you're reacting to an emotional trigger rather than to real hunger. It's a conditioned response to feelings, and you're choosing to act out with food.

Thirty-three Reasons for Self-Sabotaging

1. Anger
2. Bad timing
3. Boredom
4. Carelessness
5. Cockiness
6. Control
7. Depression
8. Envy
9. Exhaustion
10. Fear of failure
11. Fear of sexuality
12. Fear of success
13. Frustration
14. Guilt
15. Impatience
16. Intimidation
17. Jealousy
18. Lack of commitment
19. Lack of confidence
20. Lack of preparation
21. Lack of resilience
22. Lack of self-importance
23. Lack of willpower
24. Laziness
25. Loneliness
26. Neglect
27. Overcompensation
28. Self-centeredness
29. Self-deception
30. Self-destruction
31. Shame
32. Starvation
33. Stress

Emotional Eating

Hunger—the survival mechanism that tells us when to go out and hunt and forage, and how much to eat and how much to drag back to the cave—is an instinct hardwired into our gut and brain. It's a natural impulse that helped us become the magnificent creatures that we are as human beings. But today we must be careful of what we eat, and how much, and how often. Hunger can be subtle. You hardly notice being satisfied as your belly fills up with processed mush, but then the feeling of being stuffed hits you in the gut. The goal is to listen to our bodies and eat with instinct, not desire, and to know our bodies well enough to recognize when hunger has been abated.

The emotions that make us eat when we are *not* hungry are varied. Most of them start in childhood, when our parents give us a cookie because we're hurt, the doctor hands us a lollipop after getting a shot, or the school throws an ice-cream party when our team wins. Any type of celebration is connected to putting something in our mouths. Every upset is soothed with food, so that food becomes related to feelings rather than to hunger. (No wonder we have so many food issues and oral gratification problems later in life!) I wrote a lot about this in my book *Healthy Kids* because I wanted parents to become aware of this syndrome and break the cycle. It's very difficult as an adult to break it, because by then the behaviors are so ingrained in us. But in order to have the right relationship with food, the cycle must be stopped.

A good question to answer is: How did I handle my emotions as a kid? It all started there. When we want to self-sabotage, we still go back to that little kid inside us, but now we're just playing out the adult version of it. We also mirror much of what we've seen in our parents. If our parents self-medicate, or get angry, or drink too much, we'll tend to pick up some of their behaviors. We can find ourselves acting like one or both of our parents just to live in their world for a little while in order to try to understand where they're coming from. And sometimes we do the opposite of what they do, just to be sure we *don't* end up like them.

Self-sabotage is also a way of acting out. Like a spoiled child in a temper tantrum who wants what he wants when he wants it, your inner brat feels you deserve to eat everything you want, at any time you want it, without the consequences of overindulgence. But it's really a rage against one's self, because instead of being a case of "I'll show you!" it's a case of "I'll show *me*!"

Food Is Seductive

A lot of times we turn to eating because food doesn't disappoint us the way other things do. You may be upset because of the way you look or feel as a result of eating, but you're not correlating those feelings at the time of eating and tasting. Food looks good and smells good, and you *know* it's going to taste good. There's no connection, at the moment you're lusting after it, between eating something tasty and how your clothes or stomach will feel afterward. You can use anything as an excuse to eat, but the truth is you don't *need* an excuse to eat.

> Eating is fabulous!
> Eating is incredible!
> Eating is one of the greatest pleasures in life!

And it's something you get to do every day. (Can you imagine how boring it would be if you got to eat only once a week?) Our lives are so complicated, with so many different relationships, that it's no wonder we turn to food. Food doesn't talk back, and we don't have to take care of it. It takes care of us! But food is one of the most powerful relationships we have because it's really so one-sided. We place all this emotion onto food, while it is just an inanimate object with no agenda. We do all this acting out with it, and it really just sits there.

Isn't it about time we straightened out our relationship with food?

Misplaced Anger

A friend of mine was afraid to become healthy and look her best, because every time she got close to a healthy weight, it made her get in touch with her anger. She felt that getting healthy and looking good turned her into a raving bitch, and staying heavy and protected with "body armor" forced her to be sweeter to people. Being "less" than she could be, she felt beneath other people and therefore had to be *nice*. When she felt her own power because of a weight loss, she had to start working on anger issues that had been deep-rooted since childhood, and that was too much for her. It was easier to stay invisibly large (there's an oxymoron for you!) and in denial. She also couldn't handle the idea that when she looked and felt her best, other people were jealous of her. As the mother of daughters, she preferred to keep herself heavy and in the background in order to keep from competing in any way with her girls, even though they preferred her to be healthy and fit.

When I told this story to the women on Marilu.com, many of them could relate to holding themselves back so that others wouldn't get jealous or competitive. Women are conditioned in our culture to be submissive and not seek too much attention. As a result, we often feel more comfortable and unobtrusive in supporting roles. This submissiveness keeps so many of us from achieving what we want most from life. Rather than going for our dreams, we hang back and justify this self-sabotage by thinking that we're doing it for other people. When I hear stories from other women supporting this attitude, I always tell them, "This is your one chance to live the life you want and be the person you want to be! Don't fool yourself into thinking that you can't be your best because it would somehow hurt others. It's just not true!" Despite what many women think, their men want them to be fit and healthy (if not, they're with the wrong guy!) and their children want them to be vibrant, healthy people. Recognizing and overcoming the illusions that they have been buying into will be the way they conquer these feelings and will allow them to live their best lives possible.

The Power of Body Armor

When I weighed fifty-five pounds more than I do now, I used to make a lot of jokes about wearing a fat suit. I felt like the healthier, thinner me was in there somewhere, but for many stupid reasons I was choosing to insulate the thin me with body armor. Body armor is that protective layer of padding that keeps us cushioned from the outside world. When you hide yourself with body armor for a long time and then lose weight, you start to get noticed more and can no longer feel invisible. It's often too much pressure to handle, so you find ways to put the weight back on in order to go back into hiding.

Self-sabotage is also a way of filling up and isolating yourself when you think you're doing too much for other people. You get sick of giving and giving, so you overeat as a way of pulling back to protect yourself from the demands of others. Sometimes you think that if the world expects more from you, you owe the world more in return, but that's just not the case. Finally knowing what you want doesn't mean that you must abandon your desires in order to serve the demands of others. You have a responsibility to be your best only for yourself and then for the ones you love.

I know from my own experience that putting on weight can create a safe world in which to live. After you've struggled with other issues, the world of weight becomes a convenient place to go and act out. It's easier to play with that familiar little body issue "toy box" than to look at everything else in your life. Believe me, I know so much about that ten, twenty, or fifty pounds you can fool around with at the expense of everything else. It's easy to fill the time that could be better spent focusing on more important issues.

We trip ourselves up many times, over and over again, because we can. We *know* how to do it. We *know* the results our self-sabotage will bring. We *know* the convenient distraction it will be for everything else we want to do. There are many different elements to self-sabotage, and after a while they all become boring. But we still do them anyway.

Avoiding Sexuality

Packing on the body armor can also be connected to avoiding the sexual feelings and pressures that come up when you feel you can finally "present" yourself to the world. Losing weight can make you feel like a sexual creature again, and with these feelings comes a certain amount of responsibility. Sex is one of the most important ways you deal with the world. It's dangerous to layer on the body armor because you don't want to deal with your sexual self.

It's amazing the amount of sexual power a positive self-image can yield! You move differently in your body. You feel on top of your game, and you feel like you can make a presentation to the world. Nothing can stop you. But with this power comes responsibility. In becoming the best version of yourself, your desirability quotient will definitely be raised because you'll be sending off an appealing vibe to other people. This positive vibe is the essence of what we call attraction. And it's not about your breast size, the color of your hair, or the smoothness of your skin. It's about feeling good about yourself and letting the world know that you're not imprisoned by negative thoughts or self-doubt.

The power of self-control is pretty heady stuff, and when you begin to feel its strength you might think, "Oh my gosh! Who let this wild woman out?" You might get looked at in a way that makes you feel uncomfortable at first and, as crazy as it sounds, start to think that you are now going to have to give everyone everything they've ever wanted from you. Ideally, what you learn over time is how to use that "power" the right way to achieve your goals.

You can wear this newfound sexual power like a fine piece of clothing, but it's not like you have to share it with everybody. It's not as though you have become this sexy, vibrant creature and now you have to please the world. Besides, it's grandiose to think you can satisfy everyone's needs. You're coming together as a person for yourself, and this power isn't just a question of sexuality; it's also a question of the significant force you feel in becoming your best.

Jealousy

Jealousy is one of the deadly sins, and like its evil relative, gluttony, it can lead you to destruction if you let it. Jealousy was such an ugly concept in my home growing up that my mother couldn't even say the word. She would call it "J-E-A." Jealousy is an insidious virus that affects everyone and everything around it, and, more often than not, it's about the *other* person. If, in fact, you are *not* a jealous person but you find yourself feeling jealous toward someone, it's usually because they are jealous of *you*, and you are picking up on *their* feelings.

Dr. Ruth Velikovsky Sharon always says that jealousy, vindictiveness, and lack of resilience go hand in hand. I call these three qualities the Unholy Trio. If you know someone who is jealous, they are usually vindictive, and their lack of resilience means that they have difficulty getting over any little hurt or slight. Think about it. We all know people who tend to take everything as a narcissistic injury in which everything relates back to them. (As comedienne Judy Toll said, "I am the biggest piece of s★★t that the whole world revolves around!") These same people usually think that everyone is talking about them behind their backs, or secretly hoping that they'll fail. These kinds of people will help defeat your good intentions. It's important to recognize what they're up to and deal with them in an honest way. If they're family members, it's even more important to understand them and to protect your psyche from the backstabbing, vindictiveness, and their secretly hoping that *you* are the one to fail. When will the jealous people stop? The answer is never. That's why one of the most important things to learn about self-sabotage is that it's up to you. No one can hurt you the way you can hurt yourself. You can't blame others for your failures; you can't even blame your food. You can only recognize that success will be ensured if you can overcome your need for failure. Once you've become a secure, strong person, the backstabbers will become flatterers (and then you may have to protect yourself from a whole new set of problems, such as their trying to *be* you!).

It's been my experience that when a person cannot hear any sort of criticism without falling apart, it's usually because their parents lavished so much praise and attention on them as a child that they only had to breathe to get accolades. And now they expect the rest of the world to treat them that way. Unhappily for them, the rest of the world doesn't have time for such nonsense, and they find it difficult to deal with their own lack of power. They never developed the right coping skills or frustration tolerance, so they fall apart. And they usually remember their parents in a negative way, because nothing could ever be enough. Parents grow old and inevitably lose the ability to shelter their children, but these grown-up brats do not inevitably mature, and their resentment can intensify against their aged parents as they find themselves alone in the world without the skills needed to survive.

There has to be a balance. Without balance your life can swing from extreme self-gratification to extreme self-denial, and what fun is that? When you realize that taking care of yourself is not self-gratification, but rather the necessary impulse for survival and self-realization, then you can find the balance so necessary to bring about a higher quality of life.

Jealousy can also rear its ugly head in other ways. There is a woman I know who is a real baker, and every time we're in her home, I'm amazed at how fattening she makes her food. Last time we were there, she didn't serve just one dessert; there were twenty-five pastry treats loaded with sugar and dairy! She encouraged my boys to eat some of them, and they, of course, were miserable the next day. (Let's hear it for healthy palates!) But what I really noticed, while looking at family photos, was that her daughter, who is beautiful but weighs 300 pounds, was not an over-weight little girl. You can see the gradual changes in the daughter (who looks exactly like her father) in the pictures throughout the years. You definitely get the sense that the mother, who is naturally thin, may have been jealous of her little girl and probably fed her sugary treats nonstop. You could look at the photos and the desserts and the candy dishes all over the house, and the mom and the daughter and the dad, and there it was—the whole picture!

Mothers and daughters and body issues are always very connected, and it doesn't stop with food. Our father, of course, is the first male in our lives, and so much of the way we relate to him, or the way we see our parents relate to each other, shapes our relationships with men later on. I think it's very important for fathers not to come between mothers and daughters, just as it's important for mothers not to come between fathers and sons. It's difficult, I know, because as women we always see the bigger picture, and we want to supervise (snoopervise!) other people—*especially* our husbands or mates!

Self-Sabotage and PMS

In Greek mythology, Diana was the goddess of the moon. It was said that Diana hunted every night, but once a month she was forced to put down her bow and give in to the curse of womanhood. We know now that menstrual periods are not a curse, but a blessing to clear our bodies and prepare for the next month. But how we deal with PMS and our cycle can tell us much about ourselves. If we allow the monthly menstrual cycle to rob us of precious days each month, then we are allowing ourselves to be victims. If we use our cycle as an excuse to punish our bodies (or our loved ones!) then we are behaving worse than those ancient cultures that forced women out of their homes during that time of the month. It's relatively easy to avoid self-sabotaging when things are going well; the real test is when things are *not* perfect, when we are *not* feeling like ourselves.

Every month we are faced with hormonal changes that throw us off, especially if we are big meat, sugar, and dairy eaters or we give in to cravings. Before I found a healthier way of eating, I used to suffer with the worst PMS. The changes in my body and behavior every month were so pronounced that everyone around me knew when I was about to start my cycle. The writers on *Taxi*, in fact, used my PMS stories as the basis for an episode on the subject, but they gave the "condition" to Carol Kane's character rather than to mine. (PMS was funny on Simka, but scary on Elaine!)

We've become so used to having our bodies out of whack during PMS and our periods that sometimes overeating doesn't even faze us. We recognize the ebb and flow of how we feel throughout the month, so even if we're uncomfortable, we don't change our patterns. When we want to keep eating, we allow ourselves to get past the bloated feeling in order to keep going. And sometimes the lack of discomfort in stuffing our faces has nothing to do with PMS. People get so used to feeling like they have to loosen their pants after eating that they don't really think they've had a meal unless they're uncomfortable!

It's like stuffing a laundry bag, and then thinking, "What the heck, I can get a few more towels in there."

Or at least some socks.

And a T-shirt or two.

And a thong!

What Can I Get Away With?

Sometimes we self-sabotage because we want to see what we can get away with. We get sneaky, especially when we're by ourselves, and we don't think it counts. After being on a program for a while, we start looking good and people are impressed, and we think we know how to dress and get away with it. We get cocky because we feel we've done enough work, and now we can go on cruise control. We no longer want to be diligent, because it's boring—and we're thin now, right? We want to pretend we're like people who never had a weight problem or struggled with food issues, but guess what—we're not!

This realization was a real eye-opener for me. It would be easier for me to get back to 174 pounds, my heaviest weight, than it would be for someone who has never been that weight. I have no desire to go back to my old way of eating, because of the way I felt back then and how unhappy it made me, and because the taste of that food doesn't appeal to me anymore. But if I were to go back to eating that way, I would find myself at that heavier weight in no time at all. Believe me, I could do a Bridget Jones faster than Renée Zellweger!

I remember this one time years ago when I was really excited to go to a hot new comedy club. Friends of mine were appearing there, and I wanted to make a good impression. I had just moved to Los Angeles a few months earlier, and I was doing the usual rounds of auditions every actress goes through when she hits Hollywood. I had been battling with my weight and was still in the mode of losing or gaining ten to fifteen pounds in a week on some stupid diet. I went for my tight jeans first, thinking that most of my weight was usually carried in my upper body anyway, so a big shirt and tight pants would work that night. But my tight jeans wouldn't even get past my knees! I resolved to buy a scale the very next day because, obviously, the weight had crept on without my even realizing it.

I tried on pair after pair of jeans and was finally able to squeeze my thighs into my fat jeans, but even those were painfully tight (like a butcher making bratwurst)! I remember lying on my bed, trying to get the zipper up—and the zipper broke. Crying in frustration, I promised myself I'd get a grip on my weight, since I was serious about being an actress. I found two giant safety pins to hold my pants together (giving me an extra inch and a half on the waist, thank God).

So, I had the bottom of my outfit figured out. Now it was just a question of finding a top that covered not only the safety pin but also the roll of flesh hanging over it. Of course I was going to wear the tallest pair of shoes I could find to give me height and I was going to carry a big purse to put on my lap in the club to hide the overflow. The comedy club was sure to be dark, so I chose a dark sweater to cover the pants and a dark jacket over that, and I was good to go!

By the time I put on makeup, including tons of blush for fake cheekbones (I would actually draw a straight line with espresso brown eye shadow for contouring), and styled my hair half-up, half-down for a narrow look, I actually looked a lot thinner than I deserved to look that night.

So, what did I do?

I got to the club and immediately ordered ribs, onion rings, salad with blue cheese dressing, and of course a sugary sweet drink (my favorite in those days was a sloe gin fizz) to wash it all down. Why not? I had successfully(?) pulled it together one more evening and felt like I could celebrate.

I have to laugh now when I remember how much I was always trying to get away with in those prehealthy days. I used to torture myself getting ready for an event, date, or just going out with friends by trying to put together the slimmest-looking outfit I could find. And the nights that I could successfully pull it off, how did I reward myself? Not by resolving to eat like the thinner, healthier person I was longing to be, but by eating like the unhealthier, heavier person I really was.

Fear of Success (That Ugly Fear Again!)

Sometimes you self-sabotage because (and this was also a big one for me) you have this vision of what you're going to be like when you're thin, and as you get closer to it, it's not at all the way you thought it would be. Everything doesn't fall into place the way you imagined it would. You don't get the perfect job, the perfect boyfriend, and the perfect life. It's like the old, "What if I threw a party and nobody came?" You get scared because the real work has to begin. You're forced to look at a different reason than your weight for why your life isn't coming together the way you thought it would. And when that's too painful, you start to pile on the pounds again to give yourself a "safe" excuse that you can "control." Thus begins another cycle.

It's important to recognize that success is not measured by the scale in the bathroom, but by your own self-image. If you feel good about yourself, then you are successful. In the same way that anorexia is a form of self-loathing, so is overeating. As you become stronger and your self-image improves, so does your life. At that point you are ready to achieve the things you've only been dreaming about. In this sense, self-control and healthy eating are a means to find balance and happiness; a slimmer waistline is just a side benefit!

Self-Sabotage and Control

As an actress, I would always cushion myself against the blow of a bad audition or interview by having my little goodie bag of treats waiting for me in the car. It was usually salty cashews or mixed nuts, something gooey with caramel or peanut butter, and a nice, sweet carbonated drink like red cream soda. (Yikes! Those were the days.)

This one particular time, I was called to have a meeting with an important group of filmmakers who were casting for the female lead opposite an Oscar-nominated actor. In other words, the stakes were high and I wanted to do my best. It took me hours to get ready, mainly because it was right after the holidays and I had put on my requisite seven to ten pounds. But I wasn't worried, because back then not only did I know how to draw in cheekbones, I also knew how to dress thinner than I was and carry myself like a ballerina (even though the way I felt inside was less *Swan Lake* and more *Fantasia*).

As I walked into the room, I came face to face with not only a well-known director and industry heavyweights, but also a photograph of *me* on their bulletin board! The photograph was from a professional glamour shoot that I had taken after weeks of deprivation, and it had been styled by a team of hair, makeup, and wardrobe people. In other words, I was the *before*, and my picture was the *after*.

I was paralyzed by self-consciousness, and we barely talked throughout the meeting. There was no way (in my head, anyway) to live up to that damn girl on the board! I left the meeting, hit the convenience store next door, loaded up on goodies and two bottles of champagne, called my best friend, and said, "We're going for numb tonight." (I said that a lot in those days.)

We pigged out on my stash and even ordered in Chinese to wash it all down. I felt terrible the next day, of course, but at least I was feeling bad about something *I* had controlled, rather than something *they* had controlled.

I'm telling this story because it is an illustration not only of self-sabotage and control, but also of fear of living up to an image. Oh, yes, and also lack of perception, because the next day, while in my hungover, tired, and bloated state, they called and said I had the job!

Lack of Imagination

You can also self-sabotage through a lack of imagination. You may not see a desired state of health as a long-term goal or consider having a whole new relationship with food. It's easy to think, "Okay, I've been diligent, and it's paid off, and now I want to go back to the mindless cruise control of the old days." Instead of imagining your healthy future, you're seeing your diet as short-term, so when you think you've made some progress, you might easily slip back to your old ways.

B-L-A-S-T: Bored, Lonely, Angry, Starving, or Tired

In *The 30-Day Total Health Makeover*, I wrote about the acronym S-A-L-T for Starving, Angry, Lonely, and Tired, the usual triggers for emotional eating. For this book, I've updated it to B-L-A-S-T, because I have now added Bored. Boredom is one of the main catalysts for self-sabotaging, because when you have too much time on your hands, your mind tends to wander, and it has trouble focusing on what's important. As a result, you allow anything and everything—television commercials, store windows, other people's snacks—to become a visual cue. But know this: *Mindless eating establishes the metronome for an otherwise beatless life.* The problem with eating out of boredom is the same as for eating out of loneliness. No amount of food can fill the void. It isn't about the food; it's about the person. And as my mother always said when any of the six of us kids complained that we were bored, "If you're bored, you're boring!"

How to Resolve Self-Sabotage

Trying to keep from self-sabotaging is never easy. You have to learn, even before it starts, to give yourself a command and say, "NO!" If your parents had a hard time saying no to you as a child, you may be having a hard time saying no to yourself as an adult. You have to tell yourself, "I am going to stop this destructive behavior NOW." Learn to step in and be a good parent to your inner brat. You may have to do something as simple as throwing away your favorite food saboteurs, or putting them in plastic bags and hiding them someplace so that it takes being acutely aware that you're going there to get them. Give yourself a time-out and get away from the trigger while you do some-thing else for a while. If you can't take a walk or hit the treadmill, find a place you can retreat to that isn't food-related. Your bathroom, closet, garage, or kids' room is an option.

In order to stop destructive behavior before it starts, you have to take action, and sometimes that means not even taking that first bite. It might be your fault that you grabbed that first cookie or candy bar, but once you eat it, those foods have their own agenda. It makes sense that you might not want to stop once you've started. Sugar, white flour, processed foods, and even dairy products make you crave them more and more once you've indulged. Hop on that sugar/white food treadmill, and it's all over. On the other hand, natural food is more difficult to overeat. Eating a pound of candy is easy, but eating a pound of dates is not.

Write out a checklist with your own particular reasons for self-sabotaging. Print it out and highlight it for yourself. Do whatever it takes to get it into your brain. And don't forget that as you get healthy, you start to feel a sense of balance in your body *and* in your brain, helping you metabolize your newfound sanity.

I've talked a lot about self-sabotage in the books I've written and in the online chats I've given, because I was on the self-sabotage roller coaster for many years. What it finally took for me to jump off wasn't just one thing, but a combination of factors coming together. If I had to pick just one reason, however, I would have to say that after be-coming a student of health and learning so much about the power of food, my self-sabotaging ways started to feel very selfish. I knew I was capable of teaching others what I'd learned and of doing much more in my life. The only thing holding me back was keeping on the extra weight so that I couldn't make the "presentation" I wanted to make to the world. I knew that if I could get a grip and stop being so selfish within my own little cycle of weight gain and loss, I could share with others the information I had been gathering but was withholding, *even from myself.*

It's funny for me now, because after eating the way I have been for more than twenty-five years, I can size up any plate of food and know how it's going to make me feel. I know, even before I taste something, how my body will react. The healthier you eat, the better you get at knowing your body. You really do have to learn how to size up each situation. It takes listening to your body. It takes experimenting. It takes trying different things. But most of all, it takes hanging in there.

It really is one day at a time, until it becomes second nature. Any, and many, of the self-sabotage excuses can rear their ugly heads on any given day. If you're in a self-sabotaging mood, you don't care about the consequences, and if you do it often enough, the consequences are going to get you. If you do it only once in a while, however, and you really feel the "sting" of those consequences, you're going to get in that mood a lot less often.

It really is like being an alcoholic. Sometimes you have to hit rock bottom before you can cure yourself.

I know what a hot button self-sabotage is for all of us. More important, I know how hard it is to be healthy, sane, and dedicated enough to eat well, exercise every day, drink plenty of water, get enough sleep . . . yadda, yadda, yadda! I mean, even skin brushing—getting rid of the dead skin on your body—for two stinking minutes a day takes commitment! (See pages 78–79 for more information on skin brushing—it has amazing health benefits.)

None of this is easy.

Becoming healthy may be hard, especially at first, but every excruciating step of the journey is worth it. But like everything else in life, in order to be successful, you must substitute the good for the bad. Every step of the way, you have to fall in love with something *bigger* than what is in front of you.

People always ask what I did to stop self-sabotaging, and what I can tell you is this: I fell in love. I fell in love with information. I fell in love with my own power. I fell in love with feeling superior to my cravings. I fell in love with the control I had over my body and my mind. I fell in love with my ability to share what I know with others. And sometimes—in a moment of sanity—I fell in love with an apple instead of a donut. I fell in love with the way *everything* about me was changing, day by day, slowly but surely, the more and more I lived a healthy life. Most of all, I fell in love with the ability to discern at a moment's notice what's the *best* thing to do in any given situation.

It didn't happen overnight, but it happened.

Now, that's not to say that I don't have a wild, crazy, festive, indulgent meal once in a while. Nor does it mean that I don't feel every feeling I've mentioned in this chapter. But I have learned, over time, to out-create (most of the time, anyway) each potentially damaging, self-sabotaging land mine with forethought, assessment, and good sense.

You can think there's some other magic pill, but there isn't.

And I can tell you this: Until *you* decide to make something bigger and more important and more special and more satisfying than overeating, overindulging, and over-"tantrumming," you are *never* going to have what you want in life.

Food was always a big part of my life. It was the center of all things. Good times meant food, and bad times meant food. I used food for all reasons other than nourishment. I used it to cheer myself up, I used it to numb myself, I used it as a drug and often overdosed, I used it to reward myself, I used it to punish myself, I used it to keep me company, and I used it to escape. What I learned from the self-sabotage class, more than anything else, is that yes, food is powerful, but in ways I never knew. It's powerful in all the right ways.

—LAURE
LOVELACE,
Marilu.com
member

Wrapping It Up!

- You can't move forward on the game board of life if you're constantly stuck on the same space.

- We can turn our negative impulses into positive ones.

- You may be reacting to an emotional trigger rather than to real hunger.

- When we self-sabotage, we regress to that little child inside us, but now we're playing out the adult version of it.

- Self-sabotage is a way of acting out. Like a spoiled child, your inner brat feels you deserve everything without the consequences.

- People often overeat as a way to protect themselves from the demands of others.

- Being overweight can become a safe "emotional" world to live in.

- We often use extra weight as body armor to avoid dealing with our sexual self.

- Success will be ensured if you can overcome your need for failure.

- Sometimes we self-sabotage because we want to see what we can get away with.

- In order to stop destructive habits, you have to make a commitment to take action.

- Sometimes you have to hit rock bottom before you can cure yourself.

- You have to fall in love with something bigger than your cravings.

Three

LEARN TO LOVE THE FOOD THAT LOVES YOU—DETOX 101

So much has happened to me in the last ten years since I first started writing books about health, nutrition, and lifestyle. My boys have grown from babies to young adolescents. My career has taken me in many different directions and to many different places. And finally, after an amicable divorce from my sons' father, I reconnected with an old college friend who turned out to be the love of my life . . . so I married him!

It may be almost ten years since I wrote *Marilu Henner's Total Health Makeover*, but to be honest, I don't feel as if I've aged ten years. Sometimes I don't feel like I've aged at all! I feel the same as I did a decade ago, or even better. Writing this, my eighth book on health, fitness, and lifestyle, gave me a chance to relate what is the most exciting thing I have realized in the past decade—that one can slow down or even reverse the aging process by utilizing the same health principles I described in my first book.

There has been a major movement toward healthy living in this country over these past ten years. We're trying to be more careful about how we eat, what we drink, where we work, and how our families are exposed to environmental toxins. What I call "setting up your environment to win" should also include, now more than ever, "Clean up your *internal* environment and detox your body!"

The health movement has changed the way people talk about food and lifestyles. The explosion of businesses and products that cater to the healthy consumer now means that we don't have to speak of sacrifice when talking about changing our eating habits. There's a plethora of healthy foods now available in grocery stores—not to mention herbs, vitamin supplements, and healthy shampoos and cleaning products—and this creates the need for more information in order to make the best choices. I know from teaching classes at Marilu.com how important it is to share knowledge with as many people as possible. There's no reason most people can't have a healthy body into their seventies or eighties, and that should be our goal!

Obviously no one can go from fifty-five to forty-five. But certainly one can go from being a bloated, polluted forty-something to being a slim and healthy fifty-something. Or one can go from being a fat teenager to being a sleek young adult, or from overweight post-pregnancy to healthy, vibrant motherhood.

But how do you do it?

In the last ten years, I've seen the health industry grow exponentially. Everything I talked about in *Total Health Makeover* has become mainstream. Since that first book, I have seen wave after wave of fad diets crash and burn and an inexorable movement toward whole foods and a truly healthy lifestyle. But I've seen something else, too. I've seen an explosion in chronic disease and cancer. I've seen obesity rates climb to more than 30 percent and health care costs paying more for sickness than for prevention. Even people who shop exclusively in health food stores can be malnourished. Taking care of one's body by controlling what goes into it, and getting out what is harmful to it, *should* be a no-brainer. Few people today do this, but I can tell you that those who do achieve remarkable levels of health at any age.

Change Your Palate, Change Your Life!

Is this even possible? Can we actually develop a desire and passion for something besides sugary or salty or greasy foods? The answer is a resounding *yes*! It's not only possible; it's mandatory. The one thing I would most love you to take away from this book—the single most important lesson I've learned in my thirty years of studying food and health—is this:

> **Getting the healthy, fit body you've always wanted is not about measuring, weighing, or counting the calories, fats, grams, carbs, or points of the same old bad/fast/junk/crappy food.**

No matter how you slice it, or what you call it, it's still the same bad food that doesn't love your body. It's the same old food that keeps you tired, fat, full, depressed, or all of the above. Learning to love the food that loves you is the most fundamental thing you *must* learn if you are to arrive at a healthy new you.

Human beings are part of this planet that has sustained life for well over a billion years. We have a natural diet that, if followed, will result in a healthy body that is lean, strong, and fit. The problem is that, for most people, the "tastiest" foods are usually the most fattening and *un*healthy. This is based on the perception most of us grew up with after years of eating fast food and other junk foods, coupled with decades of aggressive advertising for both.

Many people talk about being addicted to desserts and fatty foods and to the extreme flavors of salt and sugar. Like it or not, we have been programmed to love junk. Our palates have been destroyed from years of extreme flavors, so much so that many of us can taste only the really salty or really sugary foods. Simple flavors from real foods seem boring to our desensitized palates. We overflavor everything, and the food industry is only too happy to help us satisfy our addiction to extreme flavors. Our taste buds are manipulated by some of the most sophisticated chemical labs in the world. The motivation for these food companies is not to nourish our bodies, but to get us to buy their chemical-filled products over and over again. Like the commercial says, "I bet you can't eat just one!"

I have learned over the years, however, that perception can change, and your palate *can* be reprogrammed. Think of how many smokers have said that they love the taste of their cigarettes, and yet the same smokers are often disgusted by cigarettes a year or so after quitting. I once loved cheese and red meat. Both repulse me now. It's difficult, but you really have to change your diet and stick with that change for a period of time that's longer than most people are willing to try. How long it actually takes depends on how addicted you are to a certain food and, more important, how much your mind is determined to adjust your taste buds. (For example, it took me less than three weeks to give up red meat, but over three months to give up dairy.) Once you get there, your palate and perception change, but it's not always an easy change. You have to take it day by day. I know from my own experience, however, that this can and will happen.

Learning to love the food that loves you simply requires you to listen to your body and use your mind to pick through the propaganda to find the food that will nourish your body, mind, and soul. A good way to start is by eating your favorite fruits and vegetables. Don't limit yourself to just one; feel free to have five or ten. Really focus and really *savor* every single bite. Experience and appreciate all the subtleties of every type you choose. I'm often surprised by the delightful complexities of something as simple as a juicy pear or a sweet mango. And perfectly steamed broccoli can actually be exciting if you only give it a chance. You're probably thinking, "This girl needs to get out more!" Actually the opposite is true. Because I eat a lot of fruits and vegetables, I have the energy to live a much fuller life than I would if I ate a heavier diet based on animal protein.

Getting Rid of the Health Robbers

The health robbers are the "takers" when it comes to your body, not the givers. Why eat junk food and fast food if they take all the life out of you? As I've described in my *Total Health Makeover* books, the big health robbers are processed foods, caffeine, sugar, red meat, dairy products, alcohol, and smoking. Most processed foods include sugar, high fructose corn syrup, red meat, dairy, and almost anything that includes caffeine. The sugar we consume is not at all natural. Granulated sugar is full of chemicals and bleached in cow bones to give it that white color. All the nutrients are boiled away in the bleaching process, leaving pure calories of fat-generating molecules. Red meat is produced in industrial feed houses, where the animals are force-fed chemically altered grains and even the remains of cows and other animals. They are loaded up with human growth hormone (HGH) and antibiotics. They are kept in filthy conditions. When slaughtered, they are traumatized to the point where their meat is full of adrenaline. Dairy products are also produced at the industrial level, with cows squeezed into small pens, tethered to their troughs, and force-fed, eating a combination of genetically engineered foods and medicines.

If it's true that you are what you eat, what do you think we become when we eat these health robbers?

The foods that give us life are the foods that are closest to living things. Many naturalists would say that seeds and sprouts contain the germ of life, and for that reason, seeds and sprouts are some of the healthiest foods to eat. Some amount of your diet should consist of raw foods, such as fruit and vegetables, to complement the cooked foods. Learning to value the simplicity and inherent goodness of the food that comes to us pure from nature is a big step toward loving the food that loves you.

Eliminating the health robbers is great for your health, but the detoxing process you'll go through as you do it may cause a healing crisis. This is nothing more than your body shedding toxins, which may manifest itself by tiredness, skin breakouts, a runny nose, or a headache. Physically, it takes about four days to get rid of the cravings from those foods. Emotionally, it can take much longer. Therefore, it is helpful to decide whether you are a turkey . . . or a weaner! Should you give up your health robbers cold turkey, or wean yourself off of them slowly? There are two different types of people; you must decide which one you are. A turkey is an all-or-nothing type who makes a resolution and finds strength in sticking with their goal. A weaner prefers to cling to their past a little bit longer as they find strength to take each baby step. Whatever floats your boat! Once you decide whether you are a turkey or a weaner, you must then decide if you will give up the bad foods all at once or eliminate them one by one. Should you first give up red meat, then dairy, then sugar? Or should you just go for it all at once? Most turkeys will want to stop eating one or go for giving up all of them, all at once. Most weaners will want to ease into it, eliminating one health robber a bit at a time and then moving on to the next challenge. I was definitely a turkey when I first started getting healthy, because I like to see what happens to your body after you've completely stopped eating a food.

Whether you are a turkey or a weaner, a key to your success in eliminating bad food is to replace it with good food as you go along. Fresh vegetables and fruits, whole grains, legumes, and most fish don't need an ingredients list, because they are what they are and can be eaten whole and unprocessed. When you choose processed foods (like cereal), be sure to read the ingredients label and make sure you can pronounce everything on it. (As I always tell my kids, "If you can't read it, you can't eat it!") Healthy foods need to be prepared; the ritual of preparation can help ease you into the detox. Vegetables should be washed to eliminate any chemicals, and smoothies take time and love to prepare properly. This activity helps in the cleansing process.

When you first give up caffeine, you may get a headache that usually lasts about four days. Most people who give up caffeine say, "I can definitely tell when I need my next cup of coffee," because their headache starts about that time of day. When you give up caffeine, the dark circles under your eyes may disappear, and your bloodshot eyes become white again. Dump the sugar, especially if you're the type to hit that three o'clock slump and pop a candy bar. Depending on how much sugar you're used to eating, you may feel a little tired, irritated, agitated, or nervous. You may even get a few pimples on your forehead, which is only the physical manifestation of the cleansing process. But with patience and time your healing crises will pass, and you'll feel better than ever.

I know from experience that getting rid of dairy can change your life. Your sinuses feel clearer, your breathing is better, and your sense of smell is a lot keener. As with sugar, people who eliminate dairy products tend to develop pimples, but this condition is only temporary. As the pimples go away, so will go the fat. Nothing is more effective in putting weight on, and keeping it on, than the consumption of dairy products. The simple elimination of cheese will go a long way toward getting you to your ideal weight.

Finally, completely eradicate red meat. If you're giving up red meat, the first thing you'll notice is how much lighter you feel. You may break out on your chin as your body works to shed the toxins, but detoxing is worth it. Don't worry about the healing crisis. Your energy will improve as your body no longer needs to work so hard at digesting dense protein. You'll get sick less often when you're not ingesting bacteria from animals that are so closely related to humans.

Get off the health robbers. You won't believe how much better you'll feel.

Food is now the tool I use to stay healthy, fit, energetic, and nourished. Food is my weapon against disease and sickness. I no longer worry about what I eat; I celebrate what I eat. I no longer feel bloated and tired after I eat; I feel satisfied, recharged, and nourished. I was thirty-five years old when I first began eating properly through THM, and couldn't tell you when the last time was that I felt healthy. Now I'm forty-two and I feel incredibly healthy.

—LAURE
LOVELACE,
Pennsylvania,
Marilu.com
member

Wet Foods versus Concentrated Foods

Do you ever feel stuffed after hitting the buffet table, or even after you eat just a small plate of food? It has less to do with the volume of food that you eat than it does with your food choices. Develop an efficient digestive system by balancing your consumption of concentrated foods with wet foods. We usually classify foods as fruits, vegetables, proteins, legumes, starches, or carbs, but we can also group foods into two more basic categories: *wet foods* and *concentrated foods.*

Wet foods are whole fruits and vegetables with a high water content. The wet foods help move along the more concentrated and processed foods in your digestive tract. Concentrated foods are heavier, denser foods like animal proteins, starches, legumes, snacks, and processed foods. They are the centerpiece of most typical American meals. We tend to overdose on concentrated foods, and that's why it's important to eat wet foods as often as possible. Starting your day with fresh fruit kick-starts your metabolism and creates a nice wet food base in your digestive system. When you prepare salads or other vegetables, don't overload them with heavy dressings and sauces, which can quickly turn a wet food into a concentrated food because of the high fat content. If you eat some raw food or vegetables throughout your day—five to nine servings is ideal—you'll lose weight, your stomach will shrink, and you'll feel lighter and cleaner because your digestive system won't be overly taxed with concentrated foods. Your stomach will thank you.

Think about how a garbage disposal works. When you put food in and turn it on, the food gets chopped up and churned but won't really dissolve and disintegrate efficiently unless you run the water as well. Your stomach works much the same way. The concentrated food you eat will get digested, but not as efficiently as when you also eat wet foods. Don't assume that drinking water with your meals does the job as well as eating wet foods. It doesn't. Wet foods stimulate the digestive juices, while water dilutes them. If you must drink with your meal, sip rather than gulp that water.

Centered Foods

The idea of "centered foods" comes from macrobiotics. Some people find the concept of macrobiotics intimidating, but it's really just an intuitive way of eating. The idea of macrobiotics is to stay in the center of the food line. The extreme foods are either contractive or expansive, based on the way you digest them and the way they make you feel. Extreme contractive foods include salty foods and animal protein. All our energy is directed inward as we digest them. Extreme expansive foods are the opposite—they draw all our energy out of us in order to digest them. Expansive foods include sugars and sweet foods, alcohol, and recreational drugs. Our bodies are always seeking balance—that's why, after a night of drinking, we may want to eat bacon and eggs to balance ourselves out; why we go back and forth between soda and chips; or why after we eat a heavy protein meal, we then crave a light, fluffy, sugary dessert. Centered foods give us balance and stop that pendulum swing from contractive to expansive and back again. Centered foods include whole grains, vegetables, and legumes. Some fruits (apples and pears, for example) are more centered than others (tropical fruits). Centered foods are plant-based. They are loaded with nutrients, and they'll keep you from eating the extreme foods.

Although I have had many health challenges lately (I'm sure due to years of unhealthy choices for the first thirty-five years of my life), I'm proud to know that I'm improving my health now and the health of my family. I'm so happy that my children will not have to suffer with all the health issues that I have experienced. This program has allowed me to change my family tree and give them the best gift of all, the gift of health.

—CINDY
RASCHKE,
Wisconsin,
Marilu.com member

The Effects of a Night of Heavy Drinking

After a night of intense drinking, everyone expects the dreaded hangover, but most people don't expect the terrible things that happen to your liver as well. It's easy to see the obvious effects of drinking (bloodshot eyes, dead skin, and puffiness), but the more long-term and damaging effects to the liver are less apparent. One of the serious problems is a depletion of vitamins and impaired absorption of nutrients, especially the B vitamins and minerals. It is easier for males to process alcohol than it is for females, so women need to be especially careful when drinking. Because it weakens your faculties and impairs your judgment, heavy drinking completely lowers your resistance to overeating—a double whammy!

The liver is the only organ that metabolizes alcohol, converting it to energy or storing it as fat. It begins by changing alcohol into a highly toxic substance called acetaldehyde, which is then converted into a nontoxic substance called acetate. Finally, the alcohol turns into carbon dioxide and water, which are easily excreted from the body. The liver metabolizes about 90 to 95 percent of the alcohol consumed, and the other 5 to 10 percent is excreted through your urine, breath, and sweat. It is best to avoid foods that are difficult to break down and ingest anyway (such as fried foods, rancid or hydrogenated fats, or drugs), but stay away from them *especially* when you are drinking.

A good rule of thumb for responsible drinking is to have no more than two drinks at a time, and no more than five drinks a week. You should also drink two glasses of water for every serving of alcohol you consume. That way you won't be dehydrated the next day and feel even worse. Also, never drink on an empty stomach, because doing so can cause the alcohol to hit you faster, thereby intoxicating you quicker than normal. You may also want to try taking L-Glutamine, an amino acid beneficial in reducing cravings for alcohol.

Another word of caution about women and alcohol: Alcohol increases your risk of breast cancer because it prevents the enzyme that fights precancer DNA changes from doing its job. That enzyme would normally correct the precancer problem, but alcohol prevents it from doing that task. One glass a day increases your risk of breast cancer by 10 percent, two glasses a day by 20 percent, three glasses a day by 40 percent, and so on, so you may want to reconsider that two-glasses-of-wine-at-dinner habit.

Helping Your Doctor Help You

We all know there is nothing more important than our health. We spend billions of dollars every year trying to get healthy. But most of us have no idea what healthy feels like. It's not enough to walk into our doctor's office and say, "Fix me!" We have to take responsibility. It's so easy to be confused these days because we don't know who to listen to when it comes to health. Western medicine? Alternative medicine? High protein? Low carbs? Low fat? Low calories? Rather than be manipulated by the latest (profit-driven) nutrition trends, HMOs, and insurance companies, let's take charge of our *own* health and well-being once and for all by understanding life's most precious gift—the human body.

In some ways we've reached the point where we no longer listen, because it seems as if we've heard it all before. Also, most of us already agree on the basics: Eat plenty of whole fruits and vegetables and unrefined grains, limit animal products, saturated fats, caffeine, and alcohol, blah, blah, blah . . . This spiel has become more familiar to us than a Hail Mary! We could recite it before every meal and call it *An Act of Restriction*.

But what's interesting is that although most of us agree on these basics, very few of us actually follow them. The typical American pattern is to forget this advice as soon as the dinner bell rings, so that we can guiltlessly enjoy our favorite comfort foods, like burgers, fries, and pizza. And when trouble arises (as it usually does) in the form of hypertension, high cholesterol, or angina, we simply take a statin, diuretic, or beta-blocker to fix it. After diagnosing and prescribing, most doctors still allow their patients to indulge—but only in *moderation,* which to most people means, "Okay, skip the bacon on my cheeseburger!"

People *refuse* to give up their comfort food, even though it is literally *killing* them! Add to this the fact that many diet and fitness authors now treat their readers like overindulged children. People no longer want to hear about *restrictions*! On more than one occasion I've read some funny (and disturbing) advice like the following:

> Here are some suggestions for incorporating fruits and vegetables into your family's menus:
>
> - Add fresh berries to pancake and waffle mixes.
> - Combine chocolate or vanilla pudding with bits of real fruit and freeze them in ice-pop molds.
> - Serve artichoke or spinach dip with tortilla chips.
> - Add chopped mushrooms and onions to your turkey burgers.

Wow! What a sacrifice! I guess some people sneak fruits and vegetables into their recipes as if they were rat poison. I know this may sound extreme, but can't we just learn to appreciate the wonderful flavors and subtleties of a luscious tangerine, a ripe strawberry, or a fresh, crisp snap pea? I'm being a bit sarcastic here, but I think it's time we all took responsibility for our health and wellness. It's too important not to. We will never reverse our current health crisis trend—soaring rates of obesity, cancer, diabetes, and cardiovascular disease—if we don't. Forget about trusting a surgeon or prescription drug to keep you or your family healthy. I firmly believe in the power of food as preventative medicine; it's the most powerful component of your own *hands-on health*!

My forty-four-year-old cousin called me recently for advice. He had failed a health assessment test because of a very high blood pressure reading of 163/102. He was told that if he didn't get his blood pressure below 140/90 by the following week, he would be required to get a doctor's note to join and use a local fitness center. He's not a smoker, but he drinks alcohol moderately and loves his coffee. I told him that he should see his doctor, but I also gave him the following regimen to follow before returning to be retested:

1. Cut out all animal products.
2. Do at least thirty minutes of moderate aerobic exercise every day.
3. Do not drink any alcohol.
4. Reduce caffeine by 50 percent (from three cups to one-and-a-half daily).
5. Eat lots of fruits and vegetables. (Adding a little olive oil and balsamic vinegar is okay.)
6. Choose brown rice, whole-wheat pasta, and other whole grains over white flours.
7. Replace breakfast muffins with unprocessed oatmeal and a light drizzle of maple syrup.

I know my cousin followed this religiously because that's the kind of guy he is. (He's a turkey!) When he commits, he goes all the way. Just *five days later*, he proudly announced that his blood pressure went from 163/102 to 123/83 on my program! This was exciting news for him, but it's also a good example of how quickly diet and exercise can change a person's body chemistry. This is not just an isolated example, either. It's typical of the results thousands of people on my Web site, Marilu.com, have gotten when they changed their diet and started exercising consistently.

The medical and pharmaceutical industries tend to downplay the role of diet and exercise as a remedy for hypertension, high cholesterol, and other diseases like cancer and diabetes. This makes perfect sense. I mean, why would these industries promote something that essentially competes with them? Keep in mind, also, that nutrition classes are not a requirement in the curriculum for most medical students. Most of them graduate with less than nine hours spent in a diet or nutrition class. And I don't mean nine "credit" hours; I'm talking about nine hours *period*! That's about the same as comedy traffic school for just *one* speeding ticket! (One day in comedy traffic school, however, does seem to *last* as long as medical school.)

Because of this deficiency in the med school curriculum, doctors tend to be arrogant about or biased against the significance of diet for combating disease. Only the hippest, best-informed physicians aggressively promote diet and exercise for the prevention of disease. (PCRM.org is a great resource.)

If you're lucky enough to find one of these doctors, stick with them! They've got *your* best interests in mind. Unfortunately, most doctors are quick to prescribe drugs instead of turning to them after seriously trying a diet and exercise regimen. Sometimes medication is, of course, the way to go—but only in *addition* to diet and exercise, and only if diet and exercise prove insufficient to solve the problem.

Most patients are all too happy to listen to their doctors and continue eating bad food, because this is what they *want* to believe. It takes discipline to change your palate and to learn to love the food that loves you back. It's so much easier to take a pill or two every day and eat whatever you want. Doctors are also reluctant to believe that diet plays the biggest role in disease prevention, because that minimizes their own importance. If we feel good and have little or no need for prescription drugs, then we don't need doctors as often. Remember what Hippocrates, the father of Western medicine, said 2,500 years ago: "Let your food be your medicine and your medicine be your food." How did our medical profession forget such good advice?

The old apple-a-day cliché is still very true, along with its companion, "An ounce of prevention is worth a pound of cure."

The Best Prescription for Your Own Hands-On Health

Here's a prescription for those of you who love to play doctor.

Keep regular tabs on the big three health indicators: blood pressure, cholesterol, and your weight/waistline/body mass index (or BMI) collectively. In order to do this, you need to get a reliable blood pressure monitor, which starts as low as thirty dollars. The upper arm cuff type is usually more reliable than the wrist or finger versions. Whether you are a man or woman, your blood pressure should be below 125/80, not 140/90 as previously thought. Experts now agree that this guideline was too lenient. Many pharmacies also offer complimentary blood pressure readings while you wait in the prescription line.

You'll also need to purchase several at-home cholesterol kits or packets for frequent testing for you and your family. The test is a little challenging at first, and you do have to prick your finger. These kits or packets will test only your total cholesterol, not your HDL/LDL ratio, but don't worry about this too much (especially if you hate math). Measuring HDL (good cholesterol) and LDL (bad cholesterol) requires a complicated test (and usually a doctor and lab), and knowing this ratio is not as significant as it was once thought. The reason is that HDL tends to go down as LDL goes down, so the ratio tends to stay relatively the same anyway. Focusing on "total cholesterol" is more important. Ideally, it should be 100 plus your age, or below 150—not 180 as previously thought, especially if you are 80 years old! Heart disease is extremely rare in people with total cholesterol below 150, regardless of their HDL/LDL ratio. Those with total cholesterol between 150 and 200 make up almost 30 percent of people with heart disease. Those with ratings over 200 make up the other 70 percent.

For your weight/waistline/BMI, all you need is a good scale and a tape measure. Your BMI gives a rough estimate of your body fat percentage, and you can find it by checking out one of the many BMI-calculating sites online, such as http://www.cdc.gov/nccdphp/dnpa/bmi/. Just plug in your weight, height, and frame size and the site will instantly calculate your BMI, which optimally should be between 19 and 25.

Apple-shaped women and potato-shaped men are at a greater risk for heart disease, cancer, and diabetes than pear-shaped women and V-shaped men. This is based on a great majority of studies done on this subject. Body shape along with obesity is a factor used to predict future disease. For women and men over forty it's not just about obesity, though—it's also about how that fat is distributed.

When women have a waistline measurement over 30 inches, the risk of heart disease doubles, and it triples when the waistline is over 38 inches. A simple way to look at this is by waist-to-hip ratio, which is determined by dividing your waistline circumference (measured at the naval) by your hip circumference (measured at the bikini line for women and pubic line for men). The lowest risk for women is a ratio of 0.72 or less (<72%). This is a good target range to aim for and to maintain. Women with the greatest risk are those with waist/hip ratios greater than 0.88 (>88%). In fact, the risk factor rises dramatically after that—as high as 300 percent! Trouble for men begins when their ratio exceeds 0.98 (>98%).

Once you've gathered all of the above figures (which shouldn't take more than a few days), you should test yourself and your family weekly in the weight/waistline/BMI categories, but only once every two or three months for cholesterol. Keep good records of your results. Anyone who is outside the healthiest parameters—especially *way* outside—will need to adjust his or her habits accordingly. Use the exercise and dietary guidelines I gave my cousin (see page 62) as a start, and adjust your own rules as you learn more about your body and what feels and works best!

Finally, I want to stress that my hands-on health recommendations are not in any way meant to replace regular visits to your physician. (They don't make at-home bypass surgery kits yet, anyway!) A good relationship with your doctor is all part of taking charge of your own health. Your doctor will probably welcome your initiative and enthusiasm! And if he or she does not appreciate your efforts, find another doctor!

I remember the exact moment I met Michael Brown. It was Friday, October 9, 1970. We were first-year students at the University of Chicago, and my dorm mate, Linda, was talking about this great guy she had met two weeks before at freshman orientation. The doorbell rang and I answered it, and Michael, with his long brown hair and blue eyes, filled the doorway. All I could think was, "Why didn't I meet him first?"

Soon we all became fast friends, and during that first year, Michael and Linda and my boyfriend Steve and I double-dated often. They even came to see me in the very first production of *Grease*, a year before the show went to Broadway! Linda and I became so close that I took her down the well-worn path to Billings Hospital to get birth control pills so she could lose her virginity to this guy! Michael and Linda broke up during our second year at U of C, and Michael and I would see each other on campus but never dared more than a "Hi."

I left school during our third year to join the First National Company of Grease and become a professional actress. Eight years passed. After living in New York and working on Broadway in several shows, I moved to California, landed my role on Taxi, and was getting married to my first husband, actor Frederic Forrest, in New Orleans. It was Friday, September 26, 1980, and I was sitting in this tiny courthouse office while Freddie stood in line for a license. All of a sudden, I looked out toward the hallway, and Michael crossed the doorway looking straight ahead. I ran out the door, screaming, "Michael! What are you doing here?"

Michael said, "I'm going around the world." (Michael had been a merchant seaman after graduation, lived in Brazil for a few years, and was then working and living in New Orleans with his wife, Mauriceia, and two daughters, Carine and Cassia.) "What are you doing here, Marilu?"

"Getting married!" I said. We talked for a while and then said our good-byes. And as he walked away down the hallway, all I kept thinking was, "How come I'm not marrying a guy like that?"

Freddie and I divorced in 1982, and I started dating director Robert Lieberman in 1985 and married him in 1990. We had two sons (Nicholas, now thirteen, and Joey, now twelve), and we separated in 2001.

In the meantime, Michael quit going to sea in 1981, returned to Brazil in 1983, and did not move back to the States until 1990, when he moved to the LA area. By then he had his two daughters and a son and had founded BrownTrout Publishers with his identical twin brother, Marc, and Marc's wife, Wendover. He was divorced from his first wife in 1994.

Five months before my divorce from Rob was finalized in 2002, a friend gave me a psychic reading for my birthday. The psychic predicted that within a year I would be with the love of my life, and his name would begin with an M, such as Mark, Michael, or Matthew. He would be a father and great with my kids, and he would be within a year of my age.

I asked the psychic, "Do I know this guy?" And he said, "If you do, you've never been with him this way before." So I dated a lot of M's, but none of them fit the description perfectly!

I'll let Michael tell the next part of the story: "In late 2002, I was living in a beach town near Los Angeles, where my family and I had been since 1990. My children were grown and had left the house, leaving me alone. I was dating at the time, but there was just no spark from anyone. A friend of mine (and Marilu's) had seen her as Roxie in *Chicago*. I got Marilu's number from him. I thought that after all of these years it was time to go back over my life and maybe find someone from the past who would fit better with me for the future. I had always liked Marilu, but she had never twinkled in my direction. In fact, I didn't think she would give me a tumble. But I thought, 'Why not? At least she might introduce me to people in a different circle.' Of course, I secretly hoped that we could finally meet in a different way and see if there was a future for us."

On February 22, 2003, twenty-two years after Michael and I had last run into each other that fateful day in New Orleans, I heard a message on my voice mail saying, "Hello, this is Mike Brown, a voice from the past, looking for Marilu Henner..."

I couldn't believe it. My heart started pounding as I listened to the message over and over again. And then I thought, "Oh my gosh! He's the M!"

Michael and I e-mailed and talked on the phone for a week before arranging a dinner on March 1. When he showed up at my house to pick me up, as he got out of his car, my first two thoughts were, "I'd forgotten how blue his eyes are," and "I've got to get him to MaryAnn for a haircut!"

Michael says: "I thought, 'So this is the Hollywood Hills, eh?'

Marilu's house has a great view, which I hoped she would show me. I first met her son Nicky, who was eight at the time. He took me on a tour around the house, which made me feel welcome. When I saw Marilu, I realized that she actually looked better than in the movies, or even than when I knew her all those years ago. I knew this was going to be an interesting evening."

The first four-and-a-half hours were a reunion dinner, where we talked about everything that we'd been through over the past twenty-two years. And the next four-and-a-half hours were a date—making out in my kitchen! Right before our first kiss, my niece Liz Carney called and said she was going into labor at that time with her son Jackson. Throughout our relationship, Michael and I have been able to look at Jackson and say, "Okay, now we're walking. Now we can say 'Hi!' Now we're going to preschool!"

Within a week, Michael and I were saying "I love you" and talking about spending the rest of our lives together. It was so obvious to everyone that this was serious that within two weeks my son Nicky said, "When, not *if*, you marry Michael, can Joey and I give you away?"

In week three of our relationship, we went to Mexico for our first "honeymoon" (as Michael called it). He then told me that he had blood in his urine but that his doctors told him not to worry. He was not alarmed at all, saying that he'd had it for two years and it had been checked out and that it was no big deal. Knowing as much as I know about the human body, I knew that it was not normal.

To make a long story short, within a few weeks, Michael was diagnosed with bladder cancer. I took him to seven different doctors all over the United States—one typical AMA doctor who wanted to do immediate surgery, and others who did enough integrative medicine to save his bladder and his life. Two months into our search for the perfect combination of Eastern and Western medicine, Michael was also diagnosed with very early stage lung cancer during a preventative

CT scan. He had had a routine chest X-ray two weeks before that had shown no abnormalities. Without the CT scan, the cancer would have gone undetected for years.

Michael proved to be a very willing patient, and he let me use him as an experiment to see if my health principles could save a person from a double shot of cancer. Along with the best of Western medicine, Michael applied the best of Eastern medicine and changed his diet, lifestyle, and mindset to beat the cancer. That first year was so hard! The doctor visits, the hospital stays, the immunotherapy for the bladder, the surgery to remove the cancerous lowest lobe of his right lung—these are not your usual first-year relationship dramas! When Michael woke from the lung surgery in November, just eight months after our first reunion dinner, he took my hand and asked me to marry him. I loved him and wanted to marry him and spend the rest of our lives together. This struggle bonded us like nothing else could. We had been through so much, in such a short period of time. Having such a history between us, being reunited this way, and then facing the trials we went through created a bond that can never fade away. Michael has now been in remission for both cancers for over four years, and his prognosis is excellent. Some of his doctors call it a miracle, but we know it's just good health and love.

Our wedding was all about our families. Michael's twin brother Marc officiated. My brother and writing partner, Lorin Henner, was our emcee. Our best man was Michael's other brother, Rob. My sister, Christal, was my maid of honor. Her nine-year-old twin sons, William and Christopher, played the cello and violin as we walked down the aisle. Our flower girls were Michael's granddaughter, Victoria, and my grandniece, Charlotte. Our ring bearers were Michael's two-year-old grandson, Lucas, and Jackson, then three-and-a-half. And, of course, Nicky and Joey gave me away!

The Danger of "Normal"

When I travel all over the country lecturing on health, nutrition, and lifestyle issues, I always talk about people's tendency, when they get sick or want to lose weight, to say, "I'll just do this special diet for a time, and then get back to normal." I firmly believe that it's not enough to change for a short period of time and then go back to normal. Normal isn't good enough anymore. Normal has to be analyzed. Normal has to be changed.

Normal is what got us into trouble in the first place!

I don't think I'm being overly dramatic when I say that normal is what's killing America. It's become the new average, when average signifies overeating, indulgence, sloth, and obesity. People get deathly ill, and then all they think about is when they can get home to their diet drink and their TV clicker. If what you're doing gives you cancer, clogs your arteries, dries out your skin, slumps your back, makes you stink, makes you itch, makes you belch, and gives you gas, then stop it . . . *now*! If that's what's normal, then don't take it back! Fight the urge and try to change in a fundamental way that can save your life, or at least your way of life. Normal is a hole that you *may* have fallen into, a nasty habit you need to give up.

We've all seen friends, relatives, and celebrities who get cancer, withstand treatments, go back to their normal lifestyles, and then bang—the cancer's back! Why? Is there something inevitable in the slow progression of terminal cancer? Or is it just that people have been reinforced in their desire to return to good old normal—the four cups of coffee a day, the meat, dairy, and sugar three times a day, the chemical junk foods, and the lazy lifestyle? Their self-defeating desire to return to normal keeps them from giving up the bad habits and cleansing their body of a lifetime of toxin buildup and, most important, of building up the immune system to help fight off disease. As the wife of a cancer survivor, I can tell you that there is another way! The way to survive cancer is to preserve and fortify your body and not give it up blindly to the knife of the surgeon. Surgery may be necessary, of course, but so, too, is the preservation of your vital organs. All the surgery in the world will not save a sick patient. And in all cases, surgery causes trauma to the body and, therefore, must be balanced with strengthening the patient's immune system.

But the greatest danger is the result of good intentions. In many cases, the family wants the patient to have the procedure and come home where everything can get back to normal—and they can all pretend nothing happened. The patient, too, wants to hurry home to go back to the former lifestyle. And more often than not, it is the stated goal of physicians to "get the patient back to normal" as soon as possible. This is viewed as the ideal, the best news a doctor can offer. And if one doctor won't operate on a disease and "fix it," then let's go to another doctor who will! It's in the hands of the patient, but the patient is often too weak to make conscious choices. Fed on hospital food, the patient just wants to get home, where the sugared cereals are still in the pantry and the ham is in the fridge. Convalescing on the couch eating pizza is not conducive to glowing health in cancer patients, but that is where many patients end up!

We have to change this "let's get back to normal!" mindset. Look how long it's taken to convince politicians that global warming is real! It's not unlike the new Food Guidelines put out in 2005, replacing the food pyramid and the confusion over how to classify macaroni and cheese. I testified at the Health and Human Services Department hearings as they finalized their report. There I saw lobbyists for the different food industries. Out of twenty-eight participants, only two people (another private citizen and I) were not on the tab of an agribusiness or trade group. There were six people from the dairy industry (one of the most powerful lobbies in Washington) and even a man from the Lard Institute (I'm not kidding) who insisted that lard was better than olive oil for the human body! There were shills for preservatives, additives, artificial colors, and packaging materials. The sugar industry was well represented, as were its rivals—the artificial sweetener guys. Although I did get up and make my points (asking for warning labels on some foods and campaigning for recommendations on water and hydration), the entire forum was not taken as seriously as I had hoped, and the results could not be swayed by one lonely voice calling out against the evils of dairy and red meat. (Even if she looked fit in a little black dress!) When the guy from the Salt Institute, bloated and red-faced, got up and insisted that there was no established medical link between salt intake and hypertension, I knew that there would not be any real change unless we change ourselves. And to change ourselves means that we have to get away from normal!

Time Can Be on Your Side

Instead of thinking of the passing years as part of some inevitable process of decay and disintegration, think instead of time as the primary agent that allows you to heal. What ages a person are the toxic burden and chemical imbalance that come from a lifetime of exposure to a polluted environment, plus emotional and physical stress. Slowing down, or even reversing, the aging process is possible, but only if you are willing to minimize your intake of toxins and work at removing accumulated toxins in your body. Time is the great gift that allows one to replace damaged cells, to eliminate toxic burden, and to heal and find vibrant health once again.

The world may be fooled by plastic surgery, but your body is not. To return to a healthier state you must give up the behaviors that wear you down and make you sick. And then you must clean out the residue of an unclean life. The cleansing process is known as detoxification, or detox for short. Detox is a simple process that has been maligned in the press as hocus-pocus. Why? Because it's such a simple and inexpensive way to better health that many companies are threatened by it.

The chemicals and pollutants that are present in our city waters help to speed up the aging process. Chlorine is added to disinfect the water, but it is a carcinogen. We may know that now, but for how many years have we been taking chlorine into our bodies and storing it as one of our lifelong toxic burdens? How do we clean this dangerous chemical out of our bodies while working to consume as few new toxins as possible? Our entire environment is polluted with toxins that eventually end up in our bodies. Mercury has been found in fish caught in the Antarctic Ocean! Lead paint in old buildings (and new toys from China!) may be linked to autism. Arsenic used in mining has now invaded the water table in many mountain towns.

The first and most important step in a detox process is the consumption of clean, rich mineral or spring water. Most of us are dehydrated, and dehydration is a major cause of bad health. Almost everything that the average American drinks each day actually increases dehydration—coffee, black tea, soft drinks, milk, and alcohol. Cutting out the consumption of these health robbers and replacing them with water, simple water, will be perhaps the most effective change you can make in your health. People should consume at least one ounce of water for each two pounds of body weight per day. (For a woman who weighs 130 pounds, that would be 65 ounces, or just over two quarts.) More water is needed if diuretics, such as alcohol, caffeine, or diet pills, are consumed. By drinking water in copious amounts, we are performing the most natural of detox actions; we are pouring water through our bodies and literally draining the toxins out. At the same time, we are draining some good things out, especially minerals. This is why it is so important to drink mineral-rich water. Mineral water will replace the minerals flushed out by the water.

The quality of tap water varies greatly across the country. New York City is famous for its good tap water, although it still contains chlorine and other chemicals. Los Angeles water, coming from hundreds of miles away, is very polluted with chemical runoff from farms. A good filter is recommended for all water entering your house, but for drinking purposes bottled water is preferable. It would be great if our country could prioritize cleaning up our drinking water—it would do so much for our environment and our health! (This was in fact one of the issues I wanted listed in the food pyramid guidelines I fought for in front of Congress.)

A properly hydrated body simply works better. The colon especially will show the benefits of hydration. As the body is lubricated, the lymphatic system drains, the colon contracts, and the skin breathes. The body is now ready to begin detox by eliminating the waste that builds up each day.

To eliminate the toxic burden of years of life in America requires a complete body detox program. Here are some basic ideas to get you started—I'll be going into much more detail in my next book!

- Colon therapy. Start by going at least once a week, then back off to every two weeks after you have had your "breakthrough" and cleaned out your gut. (This could take three months.) Check the International Association for Colon Hydrotherapy (www.i-act.org) for the name of a colon therapist. You'll know you've succeeded in your therapy when you do a "liver dump" and can see gold-colored bile going through the tube. Your therapist can point it out when it happens. It means that your liver is finally detoxing.

- To clean out your lymphatic system (the repository of all sorts of toxins that were first pumped through your liver), get lymphatic massages. Lymph nodes are like wastebaskets throughout your body. They fill up, but they often don't empty properly through the sewer of your lymphatic system, which eventually leads to the colon and out of the body. People who have lymph nodes removed in surgery (very common in cancer resections) suffer from persistent inflammation in areas of the body that are no longer served by the lymphatic system. This problem happens in all of us to some extent when our lymph nodes are compromised by clogging. Lymphatic massage therapy was developed to help people who suffer from lymphodema, and this therapy can help everyone to detox more effectively. It's especially good to have a lymphatic massage just before the colon therapy to loosen things up. Check out www.i-act.org (the International Association for Colon Hydrotherapy) to help find a good lymphatic massage therapist.

- The liver is the toxic waste treatment plant of the body. Naturally, it will get loaded up with toxins over time. Detoxing can make the function of the liver much easier, which logically should help it in the long run. By cleaning up the liver, the immune system is fortified. There are many specific therapies for detoxing the liver. These include supplements, compresses, and fasting. You can research liver cleansing online, or go to my Web site www.Marilu.com.

- The body is a wondrous web of interconnectedness. Chinese medicine teaches us that the fingers and toes are individually "wired" or related to different vital organs. Treatment based upon this insight is known as reflexology.

- Less well known is the connection between the teeth and the organs. The mouth is a wondrous organ. It is designed to let the right things in and down your throat, while somehow rejecting those things that will hurt the body. The teeth are not just exposed bone used to chew up food. They are like keys in a piano, each one linked and tuned to a particular organ. The teeth, jaw, and gums are a web of nerve connections. Was it a sadistic god who decided that our teeth should be so sensitive—so sensitive that for many people dental pain may be the worst pain they ever experience? Back a few hundred years ago, people did not eat processed food. Yes, the ox was down at the mill dragging the stone over the corn to make meal, but otherwise the food was rough. (A nice dinner might be interrupted by a stone or a twig in the soup!)

In the preindustrial age we needed sensitive teeth to tell us when the teeth were in danger. Otherwise everyone's teeth would have been broken in childhood! Bad dental health means bad health in all of its ugly forms. Plaque on the teeth is an indicator for heart disease; a botched root canal is a conduit for bacteria and viruses to go deep in the body; mercury fillings seep out of the tooth and lead to toxic poisoning. No detox program is complete without a deep cleansing of the teeth and a program to deal with the issues found in the cleaning. The mercury fillings (called silver amalgam, though the only silver is the color!) can be removed by a qualified dentist. Good dental hygiene can restore the gums to health. A healthier diet that eliminates the health robbers, that features less meat (less tearing of flesh) and less-acidic foods can minimize the wear and tear on the teeth.

- Exercise is one of the most effective methods of detox. Exercise has many benefits, specifically for cleansing the body. It speeds up the metabolism, stimulates the organs, and creates the conditions for discharge of toxins. It is essential for good health. Exercise does not need to be extreme; it just needs to be consistent. A brisk daily walk is perhaps the best form of exercise.

- Deep-tissue massage helps to push the toxins held in the skin to the surface so that they can be eliminated. Anyone who has had a good tissue massage knows the feeling when the therapist is doing the "crunchies," also known as the breaking down of tissue just under the surface. These pockets of toxins are broken up so that they can drain out the colon and lymphatic system and be eliminated forever. (What a feeling!)

- Rebounding is an effective detox practice. A rebounder is a small trampoline with a handrail. All you need to do is bounce gently up and down on the rebounder for two minutes. This stimulates the lymphatic system and greatly aids in lymphatic drainage. It is especially useful for people who cannot get enough exercise. Using a rebounder also stimulates the production of white blood cells that are key for the immune system. In fact, bouncing on the rebounder for only two minutes will triple your white blood cell count for the next hour.

- Infrared saunas can be used as a very effective long-term method of detox. The infrared rays in the sauna act directly on the fat cells in the body, where most of the toxins such as heavy metals and chemicals are stored. These fat cells are thus liquidated, with the toxins moving out through the sweat glands and the colon. The sauna gives many other therapeutic benefits, such as cleaner skin and pores, aids in sleep, and helps to control weight.

- The skin is a primary outlet for toxins leaving the body (and inlet for entering the body, unfortunately). Exfoliation is the method used to open up the pores and to allow the skin to breathe and properly dispose of waste from the body. Daily skin brushing is a great way to open up the skin. Dry, dead skin is removed. Your body sheds about two pounds of toxins a day. What better way to eliminate those toxins than through your largest organ—your skin? Skin brushing with a dry natural-bristle sauna brush opens up your pores, stimulates the lymphatic system, improves blood circulation, removes impurities, softens and beautifies your skin, allows you to sweat more evenly, alleviates skin irritations and infections, and boosts your immune system. The best way to skin brush is to use short, firm strokes in the direction of your heart. Brush every part of your body, except your face, and for women, your breasts. Make sure you give a good brush to your underarms, the back of your knees, and your inner thighs to really stimulate the lymphatic system. Do this every day before you shower or work out and you won't believe how much better you'll feel.

Time is on your side. It takes time to eliminate the toxic buildup. It takes years to get your body back to the point of cleanliness that allows for good health. As you detox, your unhealthy cells are replaced with new, clean, healthy cells. Your entire body, every cell, is replaced over a ten-year period. Settle in for the marathon. Do not get discouraged. Remember that as you eat better, exercise, detox, and seek balance both physically and emotionally, you're slowing down and even reversing the aging process. This is possible. It can be done! You have the power to accomplish this oldest of human desires.

You can be your own Fountain of Youth!

Wrapping It Up!

- The health movement has changed the way people talk about food and lifestyles.

- There has been an explosion in chronic disease and cancer.

- It takes discipline to change your palate and to learn to love the food that loves you back.

- A natural diet will result in a healthy body that is lean, strong, and fit.

- Perception can change, and your palate *can* be reprogrammed.

- The big health robbers are processed foods, caffeine, sugar, red meat, dairy products, alcohol, and smoking.

- Cows are force-fed chemically altered grains, human growth hormone (HGH), antibiotics, and the remains of other animals.

- A large portion of your diet should consist of raw foods, such as fruit and vegetables, to complement the cooked foods.

- Getting rid of dairy can change your life.

- Wet foods are fruits and vegetables with a high water content.

- Our bodies are always seeking balance.

- Centered foods are plant-based and highly nutritional and depress the urge for extreme foods.

- It is best to avoid foods that are difficult to break down.

- Never drink more than two alcoholic drinks at a time or more than five alcoholic drinks a week.

- Changing your diet can dramatically change your health!

- The medical and pharmaceutical industries tend to downplay the role of diet and exercise as a remedy for hypertension, high cholesterol, and other diseases like cancer and diabetes.

- Doctors are reluctant to believe that diet plays the biggest role in disease prevention because that·minimizes their own importance.

- Adopt a hands-on health attitude.

- Learn your blood pressure, weight, BMI, and cholesterol.

- "Normal" is what's killing America.

- Time is the great gift that allows one to replace damaged cells, to eliminate toxic burden, and to heal and find vibrant health once again.

- The world may be fooled by plastic surgery, but your body is not.

- To return to a healthier state you must give up the behaviors that wear you down and suppress the immune system.

- The chemicals and pollutants in tap water help to speed up the aging process.

- Consume at least one ounce of clean, mineral-rich water for each two pounds of body weight per day.

- A properly hydrated body works better.

- Detox is necessary to eliminate the adverse effects of years of life in America.

- Lymphatic massages clean out your repository of toxins, the lymphatic system.

- Detoxing improves function and longevity of the liver and fortifies the immune system.

- Bad dental health means bad health.

- Exercise is one of the most effective methods of detox.

- Deep-tissue massage brings toxins held in the skin to the surface of the skin so that the toxins can be eliminated through sweat.

- Exfoliation, rebounding, and infrared saunas are all very effective detox procedures.

Four

SETTING UP YOUR ENVIRONMENT TO *WIN*

When I first started out as an actress, I knew lots of struggling actors who complained about the difficulties of finding work. The actors who were most successful, on the other hand, the ones who worked regularly, were those who treated show business as a *business*. They looked at their entire career holistically and balanced their energy between being creative and being entrepreneurial. Many talented people refuse to deal with it that way. They focus more on the craft itself . . . the fun part! That's important, too, but almost not as important as the business side. It's like the old saying, "Talent is only 10 percent"—there are plenty of gifted people out there who never achieve their goals because they don't know how to package, sell, or market what they have to offer.

When you organize your auditions, classes, interviews, contacts, friends, network, and so on as a businessperson, you begin to find a consistent and more purposeful direction. When I approached my career this way, I began getting regular work that guided me toward a successful path in it. I have discovered since then that this business approach works for every aspect of life if you truly want to find direction and make tangible progress. It even works for health and fitness. In fact, it works quite well!

Think of this chapter as a business workshop for your health. Begin by looking at the whole process of dieting, health, and fitness as if you were starting your own small business, and the product you are manufacturing is a newer, fitter, healthier, better-organized, more motivated, sexier *you*.

You may want to begin this process by choosing a proud name for your company—a name that means a lot to you. Picking a name and writing out a mission statement will help every decision you make about your "business." When I asked the members at Marilu.com to do this for a January class, each of them was able to identify what they wanted to accomplish for the year. For example, a name like "No Excuses!" or "Be Ready!" tells you instantly each time you read it what your objective should be for every decision you make. Concentrate on that name every time you blow out the candles on your birthday cake and every other time you need to remind yourself about what's most important in your life.

Now, if you really were going to start your own small business, one of the first things you would do is organize for efficiency. Let's use, for example, the most basic business of all—a garage sale. It's only one notch above a lemonade stand. The best way to go about organizing for a garage sale is to assess your inventory (keep, sell, throw away), strategize your marketing (signs, ads, word of mouth), and gather your materials (labels, racks, signs) and all the other items you'll be using to most efficiently categorize, display, and sell your unwanted objects.

In the same way, the first thing you'll want to do to most efficiently develop, manufacture, and maintain a newer, fitter, healthier you is to organize your environment in a way that's most advantageous to your goals. You have to set up your environment to *win*. And the best way to do that is to make your whole environment a *health workshop*. If a factory is designed to manufacture gloves, then there is no way it will efficiently produce shirts. If your home environment is not designed and built to make you healthy, it's very unlikely that you will *be* healthy, or at least as healthy as you want to be.

If You Build It, You Will Become

The biggest problem in creating a health "factory" is that everybody's living and working space and lifestyle needs are different. It would be great if we could buy the perfect "health" kitchen from IKEA and assemble it over the weekend. Your space and situation have to be analyzed carefully and executed correctly if you truly want an environment that will function properly and last indefinitely. Depending on how organized or disorganized your living space is right now, a project like this can seem overwhelming at first. There's usually so much to do and it's difficult to know where to start.

Your Morning Routine

The process of getting healthy does not exist in a vacuum. When you go on a diet, it's not just the food in your fridge; it's also how you look at your closet, kitchen, bedroom, and everything else. In order for you to become truly healthy, the whole package has to work together. Maintaining your health is really a twenty-four-hour-a-day process, so let's start with the very first thing that starts your day—your morning routine. You can have the best intentions, the best food in your refrigerator, and your workout routine ready to go, but if you're not starting your morning with the right mindset, the whole day can get derailed. I can see with my own kids that when our morning runs smoothly, the rest of the day runs smoothly as well, and we don't have to play catch-up later on. It's like patients at a doctor's office. If the first patient is late, the whole schedule gets thrown off track. How you start your day can make or break the rest of it.

How do you wake up every day? If you had to identify your morning personality, what would it be? Do you wake up like you've been shot out of a cannon, throw yourself together, and get out the door? Do you wake up slowly and feel cheated if you can't take your time? Or do you need a giant cup of coffee to even *have* a personality?

Think about your current morning routine. Does it support the new healthy habits you're trying to create for yourself? Or is your routine holding you back? How have you organized your time, and how can you improve it? Can you easily find everything you need? What about your makeup, hair, clothing? Your bathroom? Your breakfast? Your exercising? Your kids? Good health starts first thing in the morning. It's important to figure out what's working and what isn't.

Snooze Alarm

I have no doubt that most of you enjoy having that extra few minutes that the snooze button on your alarm clock provides, but part of organizing your morning routine is assessing whether that extra sleep is biting into your preparation time. Are you losing from the snoozing? Or is more time in your bed keeping you charged up and ready to go? Maybe you press the button in the morning to make up for staying up too late the night before. If so, adjust your bedtime so you're well rested without the snooze alarm and you still have time in the morning.

Just as you know exactly where to slam your hand down to press the snooze alarm, you need to know exactly where the things you need in the morning are located. You know what is absolutely essential for you to have in order to get everything done, so consider laying those things out the night before or making a specific "morning area." It is very difficult to stay on schedule if you constantly have to look for the things you need. Think of the path you take to get everything in the morning. Is it easy and comfortable for you to move from your bed to your toothbrush to whatever your next activity is? Make sure that everything is located for optimal time management. You don't want to spend most of your morning walking across your house trying to get everything done or traipsing up and down your stairs because nothing you need is on the right floor. Better that you find another way to exercise.

Morning People

I know I'm a morning person. I like waking up, getting things done, and enjoying the little bit of "me" time I get before everyone else in the house wakes up. This is essential for me to have a good day, and I know I'm not alone in this need. However, in order to have this time in the morning, you need to make sure your lifestyle is suitable for it. First of all, if you plan on getting up early, you must make sure you are going to bed at a time that will be appropriate. You need to make sure that you're not destroying your day by undersleeping. In my book *Total Health Makeover* I devoted an entire chapter to the importance of getting a good night's sleep, because nothing can make you feel healthier, smarter, younger, and thinner. Believe it or not, a lack of sleep can make it impossible for you to lose weight and can actually promote obesity.

Setting Up Your Kitchen—To Win!

Growing up in my house in Chicago, my five siblings and I spent at least 60 percent of our time in the kitchen. In most homes, the kitchen is the center of all the traffic and chaos. And when it comes to your health, the kitchen is, without a doubt, the most important room in the house. It's where you store your food and prepare your meals and where most families dine. Because of this, it is essential that your kitchen works efficiently. I have found that the best method to create a smoothly functioning kitchen is to approach it methodically and thoughtfully.

The first step is to focus on what you want to accomplish most. Study your kitchen and imagine how you want it to look and function. Do this with pen in hand and jot down *all* your thoughts. Write down all the things you don't like about your kitchen as well. Don't be afraid to express your most trivial thoughts about this. You can always ignore them later, but sometimes it's important to get them off your chest. Here are a few suggestions to get you started:

Problems

- Everything in my kitchen is out of place. I usually can't find items I haven't used for a few months. I need a designated spot for each item so I'll always know where to locate everything.

- We're short on counter space and need to find ways to use the space more efficiently.

- The oven is too small.

- I know there are expired food products in the kitchen, but I haven't had the chance to check them and throw them away.

- I'm missing some pots and pans that would make food preparation more efficient.

- The kids have been using the kitchen for homework and other activities that should be done elsewhere.

- The counter, curtains, and cabinet doors need to be replaced or resurfaced.

- I have a difficult time cleaning up after each step of preparation.

- I need to organize my plastic storage containers so that I don't waste leftovers by covering everything in foil.

- I need a better storage location for the garbage bags.

- The dishwasher is inefficient and doesn't get things clean, so I end up washing them anyway.

- There are harmful chemicals and cleaning products on my shelves or under my sink that could be dangerous to my children and family. I need to read the warning labels and place the most dangerous products in a safe place, and childproof the cabinets.

- Family members eat junk food because it's more convenient than the fresh, natural, whole foods that are vital to optimal health. We need to create a system that makes washing, cutting, and chopping fruits and vegetables a snap—and makes cleanup easy. (There should be no excuses to grab packaged snacks or microwavable junk.)

Opportunities

- Utilize *all* available space.

- Know where everything is located.

- Have everything within reach: dishes, knives, utensils, pots, pans, oven mitts, and appliances.

- Keep cooking oils and spices cleaned and organized.

- Organize the fridge so that I can easily see the foods that have a short shelf life. I'm going to have a lot of healthy produce in the fridge, and I don't want to waste it!

- Organize and defrost the freezer. Keep plastic freezer bags handy so that I don't lose food to freezer burn.

- Organize for an efficient cleanup system. This is essential to the function of my new kitchen.

- Wean the family off junk food by surrounding them with the healthiest and freshest produce, beans, and grains.

After you spend a few days with your list, think about several of the meals you plan to prepare and what kind of cleanup procedures will be necessary. Gather the recipes of meals you've always wanted to prepare but didn't bother with because they seemed too complicated in preparation or cleanup. Pretend you're designing your kitchen to operate as a small restaurant and you need to prepare food quickly. What would you need to do to change your setup? When it comes down to it, we often take the easy route when we choose what to prepare, but if formerly exotic dishes are a snap to prepare, you'll be more likely to make them. There may be utensils you're missing that have prevented you from choosing these dishes.

For example, if you were to choose a wide variety of dishes that you've never cooked before, or if you were running a small, healthy restaurant, you might need some of the following:

- Three basic knives: chef's, serrated, and paring

- Three cutting boards: one for animal protein, one for fruits and vegetables, and one for smelly foods

- A good colander

- A steamer

- A grater

- A vegetable peeler

- Fresh and dried spices

- A Vita-Mix machine (it works with wet or dry foods and can cook or freeze foods in seconds)

Making a practical wish list like this is really the best way to get an overview of what needs to be stocked, restocked, and replaced. The vision of your future kitchen should be getting clearer now. Keep referring to this list to help you get your vision more focused and to inspire more ideas. You are now ready to take action.

My first and favorite step once I get going is to dump or move everything that doesn't belong in the kitchen. I love doing this! It feels so good to get rid of things like expired food products, junk foods, things that don't belong in a kitchen like baseballs, hangers, junk mail, hairbrushes, and stupid tchotchkes. You can already get a sense of the progress you're making as you watch space get freed up. Make this a first pass. You'll probably have to go through it again more thoroughly, but it's important to do a first pass to get things moving and free up some space. I always like to work clockwise because it gives me a sense of direction. You can easily keep track of what you've done and what you still have to do. It's important to stick with a specific and systematic order so that you can easily keep track of what you've done and haven't done.

As you move along, keep two items right beside you: a trash container and a cardboard box to place the items that belong in other rooms, such as clothes, tools, and kids' artwork. The kitchen should be reserved only for food and things connected with food. I have found some funny items over the years when I've done kitchen make-overs for friends: tennis racquets, bowling trophies, dumbbells, playing cards, you name it—even lingerie! (We all know that belongs in the glove compartment!)

Of course, what goes in the trash container junk! One of my favorite sayings is, "When in doubt, throw it out!" Make that your mantra. Don't let sentimental thoughts creep in and slow you down, especially if you have a reputation as a saver. That's probably what got you into trouble in the first place. Don't keep anything that you know is not healthy. Don't try to save money by eating something you've already bought and still want to get your money's worth from. Never try to skimp when it comes to your health, because nothing is more valuable. And never compromise your health because your kitchen is cluttered.

Once you've gotten rid of the junk and repositioned everything that was out of place, pull out your list again to reevaluate your kitchen now that there's more space to work with, which may change your final vision. It should be easier now to pick specific places for everything, but first think it through logically so you won't have to keep moving things around. My three golden rules for organization and efficiency are:

- Every item must have its own specific place.

- Every item must always be returned to its specific spot immediately after it has been used and/or cleaned.

- Never leave a room empty-handed.

As I've said, it's all about setting up your environment to win—and the kitchen is the core to a winning environment. When your kitchen is organized, you'll never again buy the same item twice because you couldn't find the first one, and you'll rarely throw away rotting food because it was buried. Explain to your family what you're trying to accomplish here. They have to realize how important this is to you *and* to them. Things need to stay in their proper place to make this work, but when the place you establish for an item makes sense, other family members will usually honor that and return it to its rightful spot, too.

Here are some final thoughts to keep in mind while you design your newly organized kitchen:

- Organize by category, so you'll always know where to find everything (dishes, silverware, plasticware, kids' items, and so on).

- Place frequently used items within easy reach.

- Place some items that are used in tandem close to each other (pot holders near the oven and stove, and so on).

- Establish a place for your utensils so they can be found easily (smaller utensils like peelers and can openers in their own space, separate from larger ones).

- Be aware of the dimensions of your refrigerator and oven, so you'll always buy the right size pans, products, and quantities.

Setting Up Your Bathroom—To Win!

After the kitchen, the most important room for taking charge of your life and health is the bathroom. According to a survey done for American Standard, the average American spends about thirty-five minutes in the bathroom each day, and that's just slightly less than 13,000 hours a year! The bathroom also happens to be the "reading room" for 42 percent of adults. As with everything else in your house, it's important to keep your bathroom clean, organized, and functional. It is an epicenter of activity, as are the kitchen and living room (albeit a different *kind* of epicenter). For some people, it's an even better escape than their own bedrooms, especially for those who have kids who enjoy constantly knocking on bedroom doors or making loud noises! Typically, the bathroom is the first place you go to in the morning and the last place you go to at night, other than your bedroom, of course. It's easy to see why it would be important to keep this area efficient and organized.

To get started, assess your bathroom as a whole. Look at it objectively, as though you were seeing it for the first time. Is it the bathroom of a winner? Open every drawer and cabinet. Define the problem areas. This could be anything from messy drawers, to broken shelves, to cracked mirrors, to damaged light fixtures. What needs work first? List everything that needs to be done and then prioritize. Include in this list the items you need but don't have. As you begin to create a winning strategy for your bathroom, decide which items you use often and figure out the most resourceful place for them to be located. Toothpaste should be by the sink, shampoo and soap near the tub and shower, makeup near a magnifying mirror, and so on. In designing a plan, think about your family unit. With whom do you share a bathroom? If you're married or living with someone, think about making a little area in the bathroom just for him or her. The same strategy should apply to yourself and your kids, if you have any.

Bathroom Cabinet

Once you've taken notes, defined your bathroom's problem areas, and designed a plan, it's time to put everything into action. Go through every one of your bathroom products. Check for dryness, smell for rancidity, and look for expiration dates, particularly on medications. (Sometimes you'll get lucky and items other than medications will have an expiration date as well, but don't count on it.) Next, wipe down *everything*—bottles, jars, shelves, and so on. Try "marrying" products to maximize space. Put harmful chemical products under the bathroom sink (or better yet, go green and get rid of those harmful chemicals), and if you have children, make sure you have a child safety lock on drawers and doors. When putting all of your products back on the shelves and in your cabinets, arrange them according to type and size.

Makeup Area

For most women, makeup is an essential part of our lives. On a bad day, it can hide your flaws and make you feel attractive, and on a good day, it can enhance your looks and make you feel sexy! So it's important to have a decent working space for your makeup area. It's also imperative to have a front-lit source of natural light and to keep the bathroom colors in the same natural tone. (No dark orange or fluorescent blue!) A good, non-warped magnifying mirror is essential, and be sure to position it at the proper angle for good posture. You can't possibly look good if you're putting on your makeup while hunched over in the dark.

As you probably already know, different types of makeup have different shelf lives. I have eye shadows I've kept for years, but mascara must be thrown out regularly. Throw out everything that has separated, changed color, or smells "off." Keep in mind the following:

1. Mascara needs to be tossed after three or four months.
2. Makeup pencils last six months to one year.
3. Lipstick is good for one or two years.
4. Blush or eye shadow is good for one or two years.

Any products you can and want to keep should be tested against your skin tone in natural light. Wipe down all jars and containers, including the inside nooks and crannies, and wipe off or sharpen the top layer of each lipstick, concealer, and pencil. Finally, start putting everything away in an organized manner. You may have to rethink the entire space and invest in extras like baskets, dividers, or storage units, but anything you can do to improve the organization and efficiency of your bathroom will pay off in the long run.

Setting Up Your Closet—To Win!

The closet is not only your storage space, it's also directly connected to your personal style and how you present yourself to the outside world. It is literally the most important place when it comes to wearing your life well. Does your closet look more like Carrie Bradshaw's or Terry Bradshaw's? Can you find everything? Does everything fit? With an organized closet, you won't be wasting precious minutes trying to figure out something to wear. That extra half hour in the morning could be spent exercising rather than trying to find something that makes you *look* thin! Begin by assessing your clutter and available space, and remove everything that is not clothing-related. Then dump or donate all of the following:

1. Any clothing you know you'll never wear.
2. Clothes you wear only on laundry day, repair day, or when house painting. (Keep one or two outfits, but not a whole wardrobe.)
3. Your fat clothes that you'll never need again.
4. Gifts you don't like but feel too guilty to give away. Give them away and make someone else happy.

Assess all accessories (bags, belts, shoes, and ties) and make four piles:

1. Keep and organize
2. Repair
3. Give away
4. Garbage

After you've relieved your poor closet of all that junk, begin organizing. Sort clothes like with like (pants, blouses, skirts, suits, shoes) in their own separate sections. If you have two of the same items, then save the better option. No one needs two faded black jackets, so keep the better one and donate the other.

Second, think about style! If you have clothes that have no shape, get rid of them. If they're from a specific era and have character, create a vintage costume section for only the best pieces. Remember, fashion is constantly changing. What was acceptable—even glamorous or sexy—one year is likely to be Goodwill chic today. Keep your style up-to-date but essentially *you*. Hold up your clothes in various lights to see what colors and designs work well with your skin tone. Try on every acceptable article of clothing, if there's time, and dump what doesn't work. When in doubt, throw it out! For shoes, place them with right forward, left backward so that you can see heel height and toe style at the same time. Make a date with the shoe repairman. It's not only satisfying to get your favorite shoes resoled and shined, it also saves you money.

Rehang all clothes with matching hangers. This isn't mandatory, but it helps with keeping your closet organized. You may also want to cover the clothes pole with plastic so that hangers slide across it more easily.

After you've finished your kitchen, bathroom, and closets, it's time to move on to the rest of the house and the rest of your environment. Here are some quick tips to help guide you:

Setting Up Your Bedroom—To Win!

Your bedroom should be a place for sleep, rest, solitude, and "cozy" time with your partner!

- Do you use your bedroom space efficiently? I'm not getting personal here; I'm talking more about the area outside the bed. Just as you did in your kitchen, get rid of everything that doesn't belong.

- Do you read or watch TV in bed before going to sleep, or just go to sleep? Are there any disturbing noises or lights that bother you?

- For those of you who are in a couple, sharing a bed with someone is usually a compromise, so make sure both parties know which side of the bed is theirs. It's also important to reach agreements on issues such as room temperature, lighting, covers/no covers, TV/no TV, and firm/not firm mattress.

One last thought: You spend at least a third of your life in bed, so don't be afraid to spend more for quality when buying a mattress, sheets, or bedding. They say you should never try to save money when buying any of the following three items: tires, shoes, and mattresses. It is very rare that you're not being supported by one of them.

Setting Up Your Garage—To Win!

The garage is an integral part of your winning environment. How many of you have a two-car garage that holds only one car? Is that other spot the parking place for your junk? De-cluttering a garage can be very rewarding, because it usually frees up tons of space to store the things that have no place in your house. So let's get started!

- How much clutter and how much available space do you have?

- Set up three or four large bins or boxes and sort the things you are going to throw out, relocate, move to storage, recycle, give away, or donate.

- Design a plan to arrange the items that will remain in the garage: auto accessories, cold/hot weather storage items, seasonal decorations/clothing, surplus cleaning supplies, lightbulbs, tools, sporting goods, gardening supplies, and whatever else is best left in the garage.

- Do you have any hazardous materials that are being stored or need to be stored? Is there room where you can safely store things like leftover paint or motor oil? Contact your local waste department to determine how to safely get rid of outdated chemical items that you're unlikely to need.

• Store all water bottles in a cool area. Water bottles exposed to heat will release dioxins, contaminating the water. Also check the expiration date on bottled water and recycle any bottles that have expired.

Setting Up Your Transportation—To Win!

Like everything else in your life, your car says a lot about you. Keep these questions in mind:

• Are you keeping your car maintained? Don't just focus on changing your oil, although that's the most important. Keep your tire pressure and fluids up to proper specifications. Your car is almost as important to keep up as your body. However, we all know plenty of guys who treat their cars a lot better!

• Is your trunk full of junk? I'm talking about your car this time, not your booty!

• How can you maximize your time while driving? Are you missing opportunities such as listening to books on tape or learning a language?

• Are you prone to road rage? If so, what are some ways to reduce stress while driving? Try to leave earlier, plan a better route, listen to calming music, and remember to breathe deeply. We discuss this in detail in chapter 9.

• If you're setting out on a long trip, do you have all of the necessary supplies both for yourself and your car? Most of these things should be in your trunk all the time for emergencies: a spare tire, extra oil, towels, a disposable camera or cell phone camera in case you need it for evidence or an accident report, warm clothes, and money.

If your environment is set up to win, you *will* win! Think about all the businesses that run smoothly and have everything in place. You automatically trust them, because you assume they operate efficiently. The opposite is true when you step inside the showroom, office, or garage of a business that is disorganized and dirty. The same thing applies to your body and your health. Your life is too important. Treat your health and life like a Fortune 500 business and be proud of the product you produce—you and your family!

Wrapping It Up!

- Treat your health as if it were a business.

- Successful businesses are well organized.

- Analyze your morning personality and ritual.

- The kitchen is the centerpiece of a winning healthy environment.

- Everything must have a specific space.

- Never compromise your health because of clutter.

- Never leave a room empty-handed.

- Your style depends on the efficiency of your closet.

- Your bedroom should be a place for sleep, rest, solitude, and sex.

- A garage can play a key role in a winning environment.

Five

THE ROLE OF YOUR LIFE

Throughout the year, I teach several online classes on lifestyle, diet, and fitness. Perhaps the biggest breakthrough class has been one based on the techniques I've learned as an actress. I call this class "The Role of Your Life."

The idea came to me when a good friend of mine, who is a gifted actress, told me that she wanted help losing weight. She had been struggling for a long time and just couldn't seem to get herself to make any progress. Appealing to the actress in her, I asked, "If a script arrived at your doorstep tomorrow morning, and the lead character was *you* at your absolute best, what would you do if you had three weeks to get ready to play her?"

She quickly said, "Oh my gosh! I would eat better, I'd exercise every day, I'd sleep more, my posture would improve, and I'd pay more attention to my hair, clothes, and makeup. I'd even stop drinking wine at night to feel better in the morning!" She always had the ability to transform herself into anyone she wanted to play as an actress.

So I thought, "If she could pretend that getting healthy was necessary for a character in a movie, instead of for her own life, would she make better choices? Why not make believe the 'healthy her' was a character in a movie?"

When most of us start a program to lose weight to be healthy and fit, our usual plan is to eat less and exercise more. A few weeks later we see and experience positive results, which makes us feel really good for a short period of time, but gradually we return to our old patterns and slip back to the weight and shape we were in before we started. This pattern is universal. The reason we perpetually fail at making long-lasting changes is that the program we set up is temporary. Even if we tell ourselves it's permanent, *unconsciously* we know it's only temporary. The transformation we go through is the by-product of a blitz rather than a lifetime transformation.

Think about the person you would most like to be—your idealized self, as it were—and approach *becoming* this person as if, like my actress friend, it were a character in a script and you were the actor cast in the part. This chapter illustrates some of the acting techniques I've used in my thirty-five years as a professional actor—and how you can use them to find a healthy, fit version of yourself.

One of the basic lessons I've learned is that *acting is the ultimate art of transformation*, and the process of that transformation comes from searching, observing, analyzing, discovering, and building a character from within. Your goal is to create the character you most want to be. After establishing a concrete image of the character and working through the exercises in this chapter, you'll then begin to act like this character. In other words, "fake it till you make it." Your idealized character and you eventually become the same person.

When you're an actor, you're always trying to be aware of your natural behavior, so that when it comes time to create a new character, you're prepared to use what you want from your own life. You also learn to figure out what you want to discard and what you may want to use from another source or person. The following exercises are designed to heighten awareness of your unconscious behavior, from the way you brush your teeth, to the food you eat, to your posture, to the clothing you choose, to how you talk to your significant other, your children, or your boss—all will be noted. You will be truly and honestly creating a character and knowing yourself well enough to do what is necessary to become the character, and for the character to become *you*.

The real fun comes from knowing that you can try on the characteristics of all types of people without having to become them. It's acceptable to test out as many as possible and then choose the ones that appeal to you. For example, if you were to "act" more fit, what would that look like? Would you stand taller? Straighter? Would you have more bounce in your step? Walk with greater purpose? These are not difficult things to do. If you try carrying yourself this way, you may find that it is easy enough to do every day and adopt it as part of your new persona.

At this point you may be thinking, "But I'm not an actor!" Don't worry. You *are* an actor. In fact, we're *all* actors. Think about it. When was the last time you had to act? Waking up in the morning when you didn't want to? Being nice to someone you couldn't stand? Going to a party when all you wanted to do was stay home in your jammies? There are always occasions when you have to act. This chapter is designed to be food for thought for what will (I hope!) develop into a soul-searching transformation. It's a road map to finding the person you know you're capable of being, not just for a short period of time, but for the rest of your long, healthy, and productive life. It's all about breaking habits. It's about becoming aware of what you do, identifying what you would *like* to do, and then figuring out how to bridge the gap. As unusual as some of the exercises might seem, this is powerful stuff. When you can get to the point where your whole body and psyche are in touch with what you want to change, then the real work can begin.

On a cellular level, our bodies are programmed with years of muscle memory. We want to change, and we make many attempts to change, but in order for that change to be long-lasting, our negative muscle memory needs to be reprogrammed. Many of the things we do in our lives are mechanical, and we can't truly make any lasting positive changes until we get in touch with those knee-jerk mechanical responses that are sabotaging our conscious efforts. The best thing to do is to read this material with an open mind and a willing spirit.

In other words . . . come to play!

Acting Healthy

It's important to do the exercises in this chapter, and all the chapters, at your own pace. You can get as detailed or as general as you like. The exercises are meant to clear your head so that you can move on to the next phase of your health journey. The purpose of the first few exercises is to bring you to a relaxed state of "neutral," so that you're not under the effects of something that happened before the moment. When you start with a clean slate, you'll be better able to move forward and begin to change your life. It's a way to "tenderize" yourself so that you can take things on in a new way. If you don't put yourself in "neutral" as an actor, then you can't "layer" on some of your character's habits.

As an actor, you're always trying to figure out what it is that you do, or need to *un*do, so that it's not part of every character you play.

For example, if you have a thick accent, either you have to get rid of that accent and bring it out occasionally when a character calls for it or you have to use it for every character. Maybe you have a way of smacking your lips when you speak or eat. Until you learn not to do it, every character you play is going to be a lip-smacker! I had to watch myself on film several times before I realized that every time I listened intently on film, as well as in real life, I furrowed my brow. I hated the way it looked on camera, so I started wearing Scotch tape across my forehead in order to stay aware of my furrowing, and it helped me break the habit.

Before starting the exercises in this chapter, it is advisable (but not mandatory) to have someone film your walking, talking, or standing from every angle so that you can see what your posture is like. Years ago, when I first started skiing, I had someone take videos as I went down the mountain. In my mind, I felt like a professional skier, but when I actually saw myself on film, I was shocked. I looked like a foosball skier! My entire body was one block! I knew I wanted to be a better skier, and that video proved that I needed to work on my form. I still may not be the Olympian I am in my head, but at least I'm not a foosball.

It's interesting to pick something as simple as brushing your teeth to examine all the mannerisms you engage in during that one little activity. I remember back in acting class when I chose it as a simple self-observation exercise. I was shocked when I realized that I always left the water on, I always leaned forward against the sink, putting all my weight on one leg, and, believe it or not, I always held my left hand up in the air like a T-Rex! As dainty as I thought I was while brushing my teeth, in reality I looked like Dino from *The Flintstones*! I still don't know why that left hand was up, but it was probably to balance my right hand, which was doing the brushing. It may also have been to ward off my siblings as a child—a popular defense. (My brother Lorin, the youngest of the six of us, still eats with his left hand up in the air, as though he is shielding his food from the rest of us!)

It's always important to pay attention to posture, because it's the first snapshot someone gets of you. Stop and think: What position are you in right now? Is there one part of your body compensating for another? It's amazing how much muscle memory we have that we're not aware of and how much our body automatically does, every day, the things we have programmed it to do.

Finding the healthy, fit person within is not as easy as you might think. It's not just about observing yourself; you need to carefully observe the people around you in many ordinary activities and circumstances, too. Pay attention to the way others carry themselves, and don't be afraid to borrow someone's "carriage" if it's one you would like to emulate. (You can even try someone's bad posture on for size, just to see how uncomfortable you can feel.)

Great posture equals great body language. With great posture you appear to be toned, balanced, and proportional, and you exude an air of confidence. And, believe it or not, you're actually getting a workout throughout your day, because your muscles are constantly reminded to be in a healthy state of tension that is actually stimulating your muscles, rather than causing stress.

Exercise 1: Finding Self with Self

The object of this first assignment is to put yourself in a relaxed, neutral state so that no matter what happens to you, your reaction to it is "fresh" as opposed to "reactive." It's important to get yourself to neutral so that you can take on a new character, which is, in this case, the character of a healthy new you. To arrive at neutral, it is best to start with knowing your own instrument, your body.

Ask yourself the following questions, and as you do, take the time to thoroughly think about each one.

How Do I Feel in My Body?

- Lie down, take a deep breath, and relax, staying perfectly still. (*I can feel that my body is tense.*)

- Starting with your toes, isolate each part of your body as you move upward to the top of your head. (*I can feel my toes. I can feel the balls of my feet. I can feel my arches, and so on.*)

- Pay attention to how each part of your body makes you feel. (*When I do this, I am aware that my right leg feels less aligned than my left, and that I need to consciously relax my right shoulder.*)

How Do My Clothes Feel?

- As an extension of my skin, how do the clothes I have chosen make me feel?

- Can I move comfortably in my clothes? Do they make me feel as if I'm hiding? Do they feel tight in the waist and legs?

- What are the clothes that make me feel most like myself? Is it the "me" I want to be?

How Old Am I?

- Choose different activities to illustrate this exercise. (*Walk across a room, lift an object, get out of bed, and so on.*)

- Think about how old you feel in your body as you do each activity. Repeat the activity as if you were eighty years old. Repeat it again as if you were eighteen.

- What do you notice about the different ways you carry yourself? How does your "age" affect your walk? Your posture? Your strength?

How Much Do I Weigh?

- Choose other activities to "feel" the weight of your body. Repeat each activity as though you were much heavier. Repeat each one again as if you were much thinner.

- What do you notice about your physical and mental state as you experience all of the different weights?

Becoming another person is not just a question of "putting something on" or "wearing a mask." It's about being aware of who you are, what you do, and the behaviors you have. It is truly and honestly about knowing yourself (the raw material you are starting with), creating the person you want to be (the healthy new you), and doing what is necessary for you to become the character (and for the character to become you).

Exercise 2: Observation

Observing other people has always been a favorite pastime of mine, and even as a child, it was something I liked to do. When you observe a lot of people and envision their life stories, you start to see the world on a more global level. You begin to realize that we all have our own insecurities, personal dramas, and body issues, and that there is so much we project to the world by the way we walk around in our skin!

This next assignment is about taking what you've learned while observing your own behavior and then applying those powers of observation to other people. Spend the day carefully noting the overall look and feeling of the people around you. Zero in on what each person needs to do to improve. Don't be afraid to be critical. (They'll never know what mark they're getting!) One of the first things you'll probably notice is how poorly most people sit. The best thing about detecting bad posture in others is that it instantly compels you to correct your own. (You're probably correcting yours right now!) Look for posture that is directly affected by poor muscle tone, excess weight, or low self-esteem. How do you feel about each stranger based on how they carry themselves?

Although you see one side of people when observing them in public, everyone has another "self" that appears only when they are alone. In acting class there was an exercise called "private moments" in which we were asked to do something in front of the class that we would normally do when alone. The students chose a wide range of activities, from putting on makeup to getting undressed—some of their most intimate actions. The point was to get comfortable doing a personal activity that you may one day be asked to do in front of forty crewmembers or an audience of two thousand. The exercise is about observing yourself first, and then trying to duplicate the most natural, automatic behavior unself-consciously in front of a group of people.

If you had to pick a private moment, which would you choose? Throughout your day, monitor yourself enough to identify something that would be difficult to do in front of people. (Closet smoker or eater, anyone?) You may be like some of the students who were uncomfortable even reading a book in front of others! This second exercise is about observing others, but for "extra credit" you may want to try a private moment in front of another person or group of people. It will make you conscious of how you behave, as well as illustrate the various options you have available to you as you create your healthy new character. As an actor, when you're working on a role, even for a ten-minute audition, it's beneficial to give your character interesting qualities so that your version of the person is memorable. Whether it's a walk, a way of standing or speaking, a certain rhythm, or a way of saying a line, directors always want to be surprised.

What makes you memorable? What do people notice first? Is it what you *want* people to remember? I really don't think any of us has a true sense of what others see when they first meet us. What's great about creating the Role of Your Life and building a character is that you're allowed to have many different parts to your personality. People would be boring if they were only glowing and positive all the time, so you definitely want to add some sizzle. Creating a new persona is fun when you find the positive traits and then discover the spicy ones as well!

If you're really game, take something you observe in others and adapt it for a period of time. Take their walk, their posture, their speech pattern, their attitude, or one of their quirks. Try it on, not so much to keep it, but to see what it's like to be someone else for a while. While building a healthier, better you, it can only help to walk like a dancer or smile like a child. At the same time, try to observe in yourself something you do that isn't necessarily attractive, something that if you saw it in a movie you would want to change, and replace it with a more desirable behavior. If you're stoop-shouldered on one side or walk with your head down, there are definite ways to improve those negative aspects of your posture.

As an actor, when you're working on a character, you usually start by using what you can from your own life as you begin to layer on the behaviors of the role. Eventually, you become emotionally and psychologically one and the same, so that you and your character become seamless. Depending on the length of the shoot or the run of the play, you learn after a while how to go back and forth between you and your character, but there are always aspects of your character that live in you while you are doing the role. I know that when I was playing Roxie Hart in the Broadway show *Chicago*, the choreographer Bob Fosse was always in my body, and it took a good year to get him out of there! Besides being trained in the Fosse technique to do my job, I also found myself adding a lot more slinky black clothing to my wardrobe and moving differently in my life. I even started wearing red lipstick, darker eye makeup, and period pieces from the 1920s. In a way, I was giving myself all the help I could to become Roxie, so that when I hit the stage, she wasn't something that I was just "putting on."

During these exercises, as you become more and more conscious of who you are and the person you want to become, you'll start to become aware of the parts of you that should stay and the parts that should go. I'm sure the people in your life won't complain, and, if anything, becoming this new healthy person should produce a positive reaction, because it's who you *really* want to be. (And if there *is* a bad reaction, then perhaps there are other issues!) Once this character is part of you it becomes second nature. Most people, unless they live with you twenty-four hours a day, won't even be aware of the subtle changes you'll be making over time. (And if you can make huge changes for the better, let them be confused!) These exercises are designed to move you closer than ever to being the person you've always wanted to be. Even if you only play the new you for a short period of time, it's a way of trying on for size the character you've always promised yourself was "in there."

This very thing happened to me when I first started therapy. I was working on the Broadway show *Grease*, and I felt that the people in the cast treated me a certain way based on the pre-analysis me. About six months into therapy, I began working on a new show, *Pal Joey*, with a completely different cast who responded differently to me than the first group did. When *Pal Joey* ended and I went back to *Grease*, it was only a matter of weeks before I was back in the same old rut with my way of interacting with that cast. Realizing this, I made drastic changes (or what felt like drastic changes at the time) in the way I related to the *Grease* people, just so they would be compelled to treat me like the new me. If I hadn't been through the experience with the *Pal Joey* gang, I never would have done what was necessary with my original group.

Because of therapy, I was definitely more confident with that second group, and that confidence manifested itself in many ways. I took more time with people; I was more in touch with my feelings and, therefore, other people's feelings. I became a better listener and more conscious of what other people were trying to say. By going through therapy and understanding better the inner workings of my mind, it was as though I had put on "X-ray" glasses that gave me better insight and more clarity than I had before going into therapy.

Taking in other people's behavior as well as your own and then analyzing where it comes from makes such a difference in the way you end up perceiving all behavior. One of my favorite stories of observation involves an athlete who was asked to mimic the movement and behavior of a two-year-old, to see what kind of workout a two-year-old gets every day in comparison with an adult athlete. Within two hours, the athlete was exhausted! If you really want to get a great workout, do whatever a two-year-old does. Another interesting exercise is to observe how people act in their cars when they are alone. Imagine all the nose-pickers and scratchers you'll catch!

Enjoy observing people, and don't feel bad about "stealing" something good (forget the nose-picking!) that works for you.

Exercise 3: Food for Thought

The third assignment is to eat a meal with your eyes closed. Get in touch with the tastes, smells, and textures of your food. Without the visual cues, observe how much you really want to eat. See if aromas, flavors, and textures become intensified because you've shut down one of your senses. This experiment is not only fun (and possibly messy!), it also helps put you in touch with the way you currently deal with food and how you want your new character to appreciate and experience food. You may discover that you barely taste the flavors, or that it's all about the visual cues for you. This exercise will make you aware of whether you rush through your meals, or how you may not be enjoying what's in front of you or listening to your body. You may find the size of your portions changing when you are unaware of the amount of food on your plate. Try this exercise several times during the day or whenever you feel you need to remind yourself to pay attention to the way you eat. This exercise will force you to take your time, because you won't be able to haphazardly "spear" at what you're eating. (You can also try this exercise blindfolded with a sexy partner, a la Kim Basinger and Micky Rourke in *9½ Weeks*, but that's more likely to lead to different discoveries!)

When I start working on a character, my mind races with questions like, "What kind of music is this character? What kind of wardrobe? What kind of material? If she were a room in her house, which one would she be?" You really want to think of your character in every way, so that she becomes a well-rounded person in your mind. You can even think of your character in terms of food; not only what she would eat, or how much, but also very specifically, as in, if she were a type of fruit, which one would she be?

The character I played in *Chicago*, Roxie, and the character I played in *Annie Get Your Gun*, Annie, are very different. Roxie is definitely a strawberry—thin-skinned and loves to be dipped in chocolate or sugar. Annie is a prickly pear. And I am definitely a cherimoya! (A cherimoya has a thick skin, many facets, softer insides, and lots of seeds for inspiration!)

You can take any category and expand it. For example, one day I thought of more than twenty food-related categories to help identify a character. Try it. Some of the answers will pop into your head instantly, and some of them you won't be able to identify right away. The goal is to think of what you are, and what your character is, and how to interpret the differences between the two.

Just for the heck of it, decide what your character and you are in the following categories: a fruit, a vegetable, a protein, a drink, a grain, a legume (peas, peanuts, lentils, soybeans, and so on), an appetizer, an entrée, a breakfast, a lunch, a dinner, a snack, china, cutlery (knife, fork, or spoon), a kitchen utensil, a condiment, a spice, a dessert, a liquor, a candy, a pasta, a side dish, a preparation of eggs, and a preparation of potato.

What kind of eater is your character? What about you? How do you eat throughout the day? Do you like to eat big meals or a lot of mini-snacks? Do you pick a little bit at everything you can find? Or are your meals the same basic foods day after day? You don't have to answer all of the questions, and they can be as simple, complicated, serious, or funny as you want them to be. This is all *literally* "food" for thought!

I'm trying to get you to expand your mind in order to see the possibilities of each category mentioned. The more options you have, the more specific you will be about your character and about yourself when choosing something from the list. You'll see how mind-bending this can be, because seeing what items you are and what items your character is (and where the choices are very similar or different) will tell you a lot about the journey you must take. When I think about the characters I've already mentioned, Roxie is definitely a spoon, Annie is a knife, and I am much more like the practical fork. (Or maybe a whisk, because I like to stir things up!)

Exercise 4: The Rant

I realized very early in life that I wanted to be an actress, and it helped me sharpen my powers of observation, not only for other people, but of course for myself. I knew that no emotion would ever be wasted. Every painful experience in my life, every slight, every hurt, and every sadness, as well as every joy and success, would help me create the characters I would portray. We often try to protect ourselves from our feelings because they are too painful, and it's much easier to be numb. We tend to insulate ourselves with food, bad habits, alcohol, and other vices.

One of the most effective exercises I've ever seen in an acting class was one where the teacher asked each of us to sit alone in the middle of the stage and vent for two minutes about someone or something that was bothering us. We were not allowed to stop talking for the entire two minutes, thereby forcing us to tap into feelings without pausing to overanalyze or become self-conscious. This exercise was called The Rant.

Either aloud or in a journal (or both!), unleash a nonstop rant for two minutes about someone or something. Direct it at your husband, mother-in-law, sister, friend, boss, or inner brat. It could also be aimed at sugar, dairy, pizza, a dead-end job, or anything else that could be sabotaging your efforts to move forward in your life. This exercise is a no-nonsense way to get in touch with what's really on your mind and perhaps hindering your progress.

There's always something to rant about, and the more you rant, the more benign your rage becomes. Sometimes the person you are ranting about is someone you desperately want to communicate with but can't, so you either harbor resentment or you turn it on yourself. Putting feelings into words gives you power over those feelings because language is powerful. If you let problems and issues intensify, you are only going to hurt yourself. The buildup will keep you from moving on or taking in anything new. You'll get frustrated faster, and holding onto the stress can cause a lot of physical problems.

One of my friends is like that. She suppresses everything. She is one of the nicest people in the world, but every once in a while she falls into what her father calls her Rumpelstiltskin mood. Like Rumpelstiltskin, who got so angry he fell through the floor, her anger is very intense and often comes out of nowhere. She's almost unrecognizable in her anger. Rather than exploding with rage, it's always better to turn on the release valve a little bit at a time so that you don't make yourself sick or fall into a depression. As Dr. Sharon always says, "Depression is anger turned inward."

One of the remarkable things about the human psyche is that we have an entire roulette wheel of emotions available to us. You could spin the wheel at any time, and it could land anywhere. It's great to have this kaleidoscope of emotions accessible at a moment's notice, and it's important that we allow ourselves to acknowledge this fact. Once a person gets in touch with his feelings and learns to understand them, he or she can judge which ones to act upon. This is why a rant is a safe environment to deal directly with your feelings.

I remember when I first did a scene in the brilliant acting teacher Ed Kaye Martin's class. It was my first time working in his class, and I went into it thinking, "He's going to be so impressed with me! I've worked on Broadway and done movies, blah, blah, blah . . . !" (So obnoxious, and so obviously scared of the new class!) I got one line out, and he busted me for being completely disconnected from the character, and who she was, and what she was saying. As he questioned my motives and characterization, I found myself weeping on stage, and in the middle of my weeping, he said, "Okay . . . start the scene."

It was not at all what I expected the scene to be, but trying it from that perspective made the character so much more real and vulnerable. I was much more in touch with her struggle and her relationship to the other character on stage. It was probably some of the best acting I ever did, and I never forgot the lesson I learned. It proved to me how typical it is to walk through your life so full of what you think you should be that you put so many masks and layers between the vulnerable person you really are inside and the person you show to the world. Ed Kaye Martin was inspiring as a teacher because he knew how to get you to the heart of your essence, find the essence of the character, and then connect the two.

The day of your rant, you may want to take a walk without your iPod, cell phone, or anything else that can distract you. Pay attention to everything around you—the sights, sounds, and smells of your world— and, especially, to the way your body moves when it follows its natural rhythm. Doing this will definitely help you work off that rant!

I loved the two-minute "rant" portion of this class. It was so releasing to just rant for two minutes straight. At the time of this class my dad had been sick and in a nursing home for ten months, and the stress I was feeling was almost unbearable. I spent two minutes writing my rant, and I felt the stress leave my body and my mind as I did it. I've used the two-minute rant in other areas of my life when I was feeling down or just bugged by others or certain situations, with the same amazing results.

—JILL NELSON,
Minnesota,
Marilu.com
member

Exercise 5: Sense Memory

This is one of my favorite acting exercises, and I've used it for every character I have ever played. The exercise is called Sense Memory, and it will help you get into a certain emotional state to achieve the results you need. In this exercise you use something, whether it is an object, image, music, or smell, to elicit a particular emotional response. The purpose of this exercise is to find a sense memory that has a powerful effect on you. You can choose one that either inspires you to feel closer to your character or softens or strengthens you to take positive action in some aspect of your life. The idea is to "spend time" with this sense memory by thinking of it, looking at it, listening to it, smelling it, and so on. If you can't think of any specific sense memory, find a photograph or something from your past when you felt your best, or pick something your character would pick. If nothing else, you can always pick a theme song for your character!

If you feel as if you have a lot of sense memories and you don't know which to choose, don't worry about it. Do any one you can. Sense memories happen throughout your day, without your even realizing it. The object of this exercise is not to pick one and then put it away. The idea is to have your emotions ready for you to use whenever you need to call on them.

Sense memory is a great exercise for teaching you how to size up something instantly and know how it will affect you. Eventually you'll get to the point, especially with food, where you'll know how badly you'll feel if you indulge—or how good you'll feel if you don't! Sense memory will help connect you to your cravings and train you to be superior to them. Put it this way: The different influences that affect you are like little magnets attached to your psyche or body, and they'll always be part of you. Making them work for you, rather than against you, is ideal.

A friend of mine tells a beautiful story about how her father always kept a certain type of cookie in their home when she was growing up. She loved to buy them and keep them in her house, and that's wonderful. We don't want to lose those sentimental gems that take us back to people we love or to a different time. But if every time my friend saw those cookies she remembered her father and then ate a bag of those cookies, she would definitely be misusing her sense memory by letting her sense memory create somewhat destructive behavior in herself.

It's good to become emotionally available, because it means that you're a sensitive human being. These exercises are designed to help you understand and be able to control your emotions, not to the extent that they don't exist, but rather to learn to use them wisely. Understanding where your emotions are coming from and being able to feel those feelings without constantly losing control is the goal, and becoming a good "sizer-upper" is definitely an asset. This is not only about food, of course. If you are able to evaluate a heated situation with a loved one before it gets too hot, you may pull back and ask yourself, "If I lose it over this issue, what's going to happen? How can I be a more effective communicator so that my point is heard without devastating the other person?" Feeling your feelings, getting overly emotional about them, and then losing all control will only kill your cause. Who wants to watch that performance, anyway? If you can find a better way to get your point across so that your "audience" (husband/kids/boss) can hear you, then you'll be much more effective in your daily life. Otherwise you're always putting your feelings into action, and if we all did that, the world would be a mess. (And most husbands would be dead!) Of course, remaining emotionally available without losing control or being overwhelmed by your memories and reactions takes practice, so look for opportunities to do the Sense Memory exercise in different situations in your daily life.

Using sense memories can help in all facets of your life. Years ago, I was living with my boyfriend Lloyd, and we were heading for a huge fight. For a sense memory, I looked at a photograph of him as a six-year-old boy on monkey bars. This little boy was so sweet and vulnerable, and so open and loving, and he looked nothing at all like Lloyd whose face had matured into a more angular, severe, and defensive demeanor. He was a really tough nut to crack, but I loved him, and I knew that the little boy still existed within him. I also knew that, as upset as I was, if I confronted him and took a defensive tone, we would get nowhere. So as part of a class exercise, I studied that childhood picture and began to really weep for what was lost in him, what I wanted to see in him again, and, most of all, what I felt was happening between us. Studying that picture put me in a state of emotional readiness, so that when I confronted him later, I was coming from a loving place. It was a huge turning point in our relationship.

Another sense memory example comes from when I was doing the television movie *My Son Is Innocent* years ago. My boys were three months and twenty-one months old at the time, and my character was fighting to get her fifteen-year-old son out of jail. He had been unjustly accused of attacking a neighbor, and there was a scene in which I get the news and immediately burst into tears. Because of the location, it was going to be a long night with many takes, and I knew that I had to nail the emotion each time. I chose to wear a sweater in the scene, and I put one of Nicky's sock in my left pocket and one of Joey's in my right. All I had to do was know those little socks were there, or once in a while, touch my pocket, and the tears came running out. To this day when I think about it, I still want to cry.

Exercise 6: Character Development

After all the difficult internal work of digging deep into your psyche, you now get to have some fun! You've been creating this whole new person, and now you get to live in her world for a while. You should already have a pretty good idea of who she is, but just to be sure, you need to add some layers to her personality and physical characteristics. Think about how your character dresses, moves, and talks. Imagine how she eats—not just what, but how often, how much, and at what pace. What colors does she tend to wear? What style? List whatever you want about your character so that she becomes real to you. And then, choose one thing today to do as she would do it.

To understand how she behaves in any given circumstance, start by giving her a situation that defines her character—her big scene, as it were. (Think Shirley MacLaine in the hospital scene in *Terms of Endearment*, Scarlett O'Hara in her "I'll never go hungry again!" scene, Sally Field as Norma Rae holding up the sign, *Chicago*'s Roxie Hart singing "Roxie.") This is challenging, but very effective. You can always begin this exercise by thinking of your own life and describing a moment that epitomizes *you*. For example, think of a scene you wish you'd handled differently, and make that your character's scene. What do you want to say to the world? Every day you should decide your mission statement, and if each day you want to say the same thing, and your life isn't saying it, then maybe *that* has to be addressed.

Have fun. Don't overthink it. And use your instincts.

This assignment may seem a little out there, but it's a blast to think about even if you can't decide on one scene that defines your life. It's also a great idea to write down your character's desired traits and take a glance at them before you start your day. As an actress, you have a script, and you review that script many times before you go on stage.

Even during the run of a play you reread the script just to refresh your brain and see the lines in a different way than you may have interpreted them during the rehearsal period. You can make this exercise as complex or as simple as you want it to be. The main purpose of this exercise is to create a specific example of your character's behavior. You can't really know a character until you give him or her something to do. Creating a scene is a mental exercise that crafts an actual situation for your character to "play."

Let's say the "real you" had a "scene" where you fought with your husband or boyfriend, and you didn't handle it well because it turned into a lot of button-pushing. Neither of you got what you wanted, and you both ended up miserable as a result. You could now imagine that your character had a fight with her husband or boyfriend and that she was able to take some of the tension out of the room by speaking more calmly and by sitting next to him during the argument rather than sitting across from him, the more confrontational position. "She" did not take any of his button-pushing personally, but instead was able to hear what he had to say and kept from making inflammatory remarks. This is an example of looking at something you did in the past that didn't go well and correcting it as your character. (I use the argument incident because I've been there!) If the exercise is too difficult for you to do, don't worry. Skip it for now and catch up with it later. It will still be seeping into your brain, and at some point you'll think, "Oh, that's what she was talking about!"

This is a great exercise when it comes to dealing with families. As we all know, families can make you crazy! In our big family of six kids, two of our nieces are old enough to be sisters, so it really feels like eight kids. The eight of us have different ways of confronting situations, recovering from altercations, letting things go, and moving on. People who allow things to fester, before or after an incident, are usually the ones who make themselves sick. Some people can't stop from letting things eat away at them. If that's your style, just go back to The Rant. If it's someone you love carrying a grudge, help them find some way to get rid of the charge, and recognize that it's just their letting off steam. I always think that the people who live in a constant state of anger are only punishing themselves. (Who wants to walk around with that energy?)

Families are tough, no question about it, and it's funny how any combination of two people makes its own "cocktail." (Some are like Shirley Temples, and some are of the Molotov variety!) Quite often family members will try to convert you from your new character back to the old one they knew so well.

It's important to look at this topic through the prism of family life, because it opens your eyes as to how many different characters you play when you're with different people. I have a completely different relationship with every member of my family, as I'm sure everyone does. I'm always me, of course, as you are always you, but the different people we encounter bring out different personality traits. We tend to want to hang out with the people who bring out the traits we like best in ourselves.

Changing ourselves really shifts the people and the weight of the pieces in the mobile we call our lives. That's what all of this character study is about—finding different ways to see our familiar situations. It's natural for each person to have his or her own agenda, and once you really understand that, you become a much more forgiving person because you stop taking things personally. People need their agenda in order to survive if they don't yet know what to replace it with.

When you're working on your scenes, remember that the most interesting scenes always have conflict and strong points of view. My acting teacher would watch a scene, and there would be a perfect moment for an actor to respond in some way, but the actor on stage wouldn't follow through. My teacher would immediately stop the scene and say, "You missed your cue for passion." What he meant was that someone let the ball drop and didn't take action. If you really think about it, how many times in our day does that happen? A small window of opportunity goes by when magic could have happened, but the cue for passion was missed. It's a great phrase, and one I think about all the time. I try to live by it as much as I can, and it really makes a difference, because those ripe moments don't happen that often.

Exercise 7: Finding Your Objective

When working on a scene, an actor must ask, "What is my objective in this scene? What does my character *want*?" Once that question is answered, the rest of the scene can be viewed through that filter, and it becomes an easier scene to play. Someone who has a specific purpose in a scene is more compelling to watch than someone who is merely reacting and behaving. This is also true for everyday life. Objectives are reached by having focus, purpose, and direction. When you have these in mind, your life automatically becomes more interesting and important. In this exercise, you specifically define your objective in each of your activities throughout the day. This will not only help keep you aware of your intentions, it will also help reveal any unconsciously hidden agendas that may be sabotaging your goals.

It is important to recognize the difference between an *objective* and a *goal*. A goal can be about one definite target, or it can be vague and varied like a to-do list. An objective is a more specific state of mind.

Let's say that at the beginning of the year you say to yourself, "My goal is to lose ten pounds." There are many healthy and unhealthy ways you can do that, but let's say that your *objective* is to be the healthiest you've ever been. Chances are that the ten pounds will come off *and* other healthy benefits will fall into place. Your goal is more physical, whereas your objective is more psychological, and even more powerful, because it's about an intention that informs every decision you make.

Many times we fail at reaching our goals because our *objective* isn't strong, specific, calculated, or psychological enough to hit the target. We all have little goals, big goals, and great goals, but good intentions alone aren't enough to carry them to fruition. Encourage yourself to think of goals that are the results of actions, and to set the course for your objectives psychologically. Gather information and learn everything you can about your goal or objective before you set it.

You can start by specifically defining your objective in each activity throughout your day. As you shop at the supermarket, think about what matters most as you choose what goes in your cart—health or convenience? Or ask yourself before calling a friend, "What's the main reason I'm calling?" While spending time with your kids, evaluate what's more important, their company or their homework. By defining your objectives, you'll be more conscious of what works and what doesn't in your everyday life.

Exercise 8: Props and Costumes

An actor needs his circumstances and surroundings to be detailed and specific. The more specific an actor makes his character's back-story, goals, motivations, and physical surroundings, the more equipped he'll be to breathe life into that character. Legendary actor and teacher Uta Hagen always instructed her students to work with a lot of props and activities in order to help them find a specific physical and emotional life. She felt that having to pantomime any action was a distraction away from really thinking and, therefore, "living" on stage. She never wanted her acting students to be without the tools necessary for them to create "real" life on stage. That is why you could always spot Uta Hagen's students in New York by the huge prop-filled duffle bags they were schlepping as they left the 14th Street subway stop in the Village.

In the same way, you need all the props that will bring the "new you" to life. It's important to equip yourself with all that is necessary to living a healthy life. Make a wish list of everything you need to make your character "live." Think of everything she needs in terms of clothes, exercise equipment, kitchen supplies, work paraphernalia, and so on. It doesn't matter if it's totally out there, or whether or not you can easily obtain it. You don't have to rush out and actually buy a lot of health food products, workout clothes, and exercise equipment without thinking it through. You're a work in progress, so the list will change over time. An actor doesn't just arbitrarily fold laundry in a scene just to have some physical life. She must design her activity in the scene based on what is specific to the character's needs and desires at the time, but only after carefully analyzing and building her character's life history and persona from the inside out.

Give yourself permission to try on another character, and see how it feels. It's been my experience that people get into acting for one of two reasons—either because they want to extend their personalities, or because they enjoy being someone they're not. (I'm definitely the former!) Those who want to act as an extension of themselves start with characters that are similar to their persona and add different elements on top of that. My first husband, Frederic Forrest, was the second type of actor. He completely immersed himself in a character to the point where the real Freddie didn't exist! We first met when I screen-tested opposite him for the film *Hammett*, and he looked *exactly* like Hammett, down to the white hair, gaunt physique, and chain-smoking. By the time we got married eight months later, he was already into his next movie (*One from the Heart*) and character. Hank was a junk man from Vegas who was twenty-five pounds heavier than Hammett because Freddie took literally a line that described Hank as looking like an egg. Whenever we fought, I told him that I had fallen in love with Hammett, but I married Hank! During our short marriage, I watched him turn into seven different characters!

When you read a role for the first time, the character often feels far away from the person you are. You think, "How can I ever play this part?" Slowly, you and your character begin to morph into each other, and you begin to understand what gives your character life. What usually happens in day-to-day living is that the world creates a character *for* you. This sometimes suppresses the person you really want to be. The whole world responds to the character that's been created over time by other forces such as choices, hardships, other people, your parents, and your environment. Before you know it, you can be far away from that other person inside you . . . the real you. It is important to give yourself permission to be daring and go to the other side for a little while. It gives you a glimpse of what's possible if you're willing to dig your way out and let the chips fall where they may.

Once you get your character on the right track, it becomes easier to play any "scene" from her new point of view. As in any long-running television show where the characters change over time, you have a run-of-the-play contract in your "show," so your character can evolve in terms of looks and personality as long as you keep working on her. When building a character, it's important to add the physical and tangible qualities that are most in sync with what the character is trying to project to the world. What are you trying to convey to your "audience"? It is imperative that you take the steps necessary to start looking like and behaving like the new person you want to be.

The great thing about wardrobe is that it instantly tells the audience who people are, where they're from, and, more often than not, their situation in life. Let's say a character starts as a repressed woman, all buttoned up in blacks and grays, with severe lines and a more rigid style of clothing. These clothes would affect her behavior, making her walk in an uptight way, sit ramrod straight, and remain rather closed off. The audience wouldn't know what was happening, but they would watch as the character's clothing changes. Let's say it begins to loosen up as the character does. Her choices become more colorful, more sensuous, and more open, and even if the changes are subtle and gradual, the audience feels the difference.

Keeping this in mind, take the time to size up your present situation. Figure out what's appropriate for your setting and your story. Think back to the first exercise. How does your current wardrobe make you feel? Decide what kind of statement you want to make. What colors work well with your skin tone? Maybe you want to stand out with a vibrant red, orange, or yellow, or maybe you prefer a more subtle color to keep you the focus, such as black, blue, or gray. What fabrics and styles help you move in your body the way you want to move? When choosing something to wear, figure out what impact it will have.

And you thought an actor's only job was to learn his lines and not bump into the furniture!

Exercise 9: Light of Day

Step into the future! Spend the entire day as the "you" of the future.

Are you ready to meet her yet? What kind of breakfast is she going to eat? What kinds of plans will she make? How will she interact with coworkers? How will she talk to her friends, family, spouse, boyfriend, or a secret crush? Don't tell anyone what you're doing. You're the only one who has to know. But pay close attention to how others respond to the future you. The more you practice being in character, the more you *become* your character. The current "you" becomes her back-story. So, even if you slip into the current you, you can say to yourself, "Oh, that's the old me, and I like the new me better!" If you really commit to it, you can convince people that you're someone different. Believe me, I've worked with actors who were so in character throughout filming that I never really knew who they were in real life!

Years ago, I did a film with Doug Savant (*Melrose Place*, *Desperate Housewives*) in which he played a killer who stalks me for years before brutally attacking me. During the Toronto shoot he spoke with his character's Alabama accent, never socialized with me, never went to any cast dinners, never even talked to me on the set. He was in character the whole time, and to this day I don't feel as if I ever really met him. And his character was so convincing, I think he's still after me!

Consider going food shopping as your character, choosing only the items *she* likes to eat. Go to a restaurant and order the way she orders. Go clothes shopping to pick out the kinds of clothes the future you will be buying—and in your future sizes! You could be a fashion stylist shopping for a client. Don't try anything on or make any purchases yet. You'll be doing that later. Explore the possibilities and how those possibilities make you feel. All you're doing is trying on the future "you" to see how she "feels" so far!

Don't limit this exercise to shopping. This could also be a day spent researching her lifestyle. Is there something you've been dreaming about accomplishing, but you never actually designed a plan of action? Write down what you need to do to make it come true, and then make a promise to put it into action.

These plans are about the future you. Later, you can return to the present you, but for the moment it is a chance to learn something by peeking into the future. It may reveal where you truly want to go.

The "Role of Your Life" was both fun and an eye opener for me, someone who gets caught up with the mundane activities of life and needs a little prompting to explore the hidden side of the interesting person I ignore.

—FAITH WAIT,
Pennsylvania,
Marilu.com
member

I loved the Role of Your Life class. I keep my description of my character nearby for inspiration and a reminder of who I strive to be on a daily basis: "a healthy, vibrant, energetic, charismatic, sexy woman." The Role of Your Life class was a creative, innovative way for each of us to individualize THM and focus on our needs. For example, my greatest health robber is stress, and stress sabotages all the ways I take care of myself (eating well, exercising). My character is a reminder that I have the power to transcend my self-imposed obstacles. As my character, "I am courageous, fearless, and face all anxieties head-on. I live my life healthy and in joy and love. I am a mentor to younger women. I am creative. I am a free spirit who is willing to say no to things I don't want to do, and yes to things that I do. I am open to possibilities and opportunities. I follow my intuition."

—CAROL
MELNICK,
Illinois,
Marilu.com
member

Sometimes we get our best perspective by stepping back a bit; it's much easier to see what's wrong with your friends than to see clearly what's wrong with yourself. Using actors' techniques is a great opportunity to step outside yourself and look in. You may discover some things about yourself that have been subconsciously buried for years.

Dig deep in your exploration and enjoy playing your part. After all, this truly *is* the role of your life!

Wrapping It Up!

- The "healthy you" is a character you were meant to play.

- Acting is the ultimate art of transformation.

- Positive, lasting changes are impossible until we become conscious of our mechanical responses.

- Great posture equals great body language.

- The goal is to understand where your emotions are coming from and feel them.

- Sense memories can help in all facets of your life.

- Decide every day what you want to say to the world, and then find some way to say it.

- Allowing the negative to fester builds an internal environment that breeds illness.

- The most interesting scenes are the ones with profound conflict.

- We often fail to reach our goals because our *objective* isn't specific or strong enough.

- It's important to equip yourself with all that is necessary to living a healthy life.

- Once you get your character on the right track, it becomes easier to play any "scene" from the new point of view.

- Wardrobe instantly telegraphs who someone is, where they're from, and, more often than not, their situation in life.

- Step into the future! Spend the entire day as the "you" of the future.

Six

RADAR, RESILIENCE, PLAN B, AND TEFLON

A key ingredient to wearing your life well is mastering the skill of interacting with other people and learning how to read a room. You also need to develop resilience so that you won't get easily crushed or derailed by what others say about you. I call this your personal Teflon. This all comes with observation and experience.

You can't develop a dynamic personality at home alone in your basement; it can only be developed while interacting with other people. Just like Hillary Clinton's recipe for raising a child, it also takes a village to develop a strong personality. It's very similar to the way a comedian develops a stand-up routine. He doesn't spend months alone writing jokes and then finally emerge one day to perform his twenty-minute set at the Improv. Of course not! He writes one or two jokes a day and continually tries them out on an audience to observe their reaction. He then rewrites and polishes each joke until he gets the reaction he wants. So, actually, the audience writes his routine with him. Almost the entire routine is based on audience response.

Your personality in life is just the same, or at least should be, if you want to be engaging, interesting, and effective. You should learn to factor in the feedback that you get from the people around you. Unfortunately, many people tweak their personality based only on the feedback they give *themselves*.

While working on this chapter, I happened to observe friends at my son Joey's birthday party, and I noticed how they handled themselves while socializing. It's especially interesting to watch how people enter a party. Some have an agenda and some don't. Some are very comfortable to be there, and some would have preferred to stay home. As I watched people enter the room, it was fascinating to note that the whole dynamic of the party changed as each new person was added to the group. I've enjoyed observing this at the parties I've attended over the years—I've even developed categories for all the different party personality types:

The Swizzle Stick. This is often the host. He or she keeps the ball rolling, stirs the pot, spices the conversation, and tends to oversee the whole party.

The Helper. This person is my favorite—the most important person to invite to any party. She reads the situation and jumps right in to help wherever she is needed most. If your party starts at seven, tell *her* it starts at six, and when she arrives at the door, swap out her Kendall Jackson with a bottle of Windex! I love the Helper! Please don't ever change!

The Hurricane. Often named Windy or Stormy! Everyone knows when *she* arrives. She talks loudly and makes a grand entrance. Some people are naturally drawn to her, while others head for the hills. She likes to stir the conversation like the Swizzle Stick, but prefers to use a blender.

The Analyst. You'll find this guy sitting in the corner next to the couch waiting for his next "patient." He tends to ask questions like, "And how does that make you *feel*?" "What *occurs* to you?" or "Give me three adjectives to describe how angry you felt when he did that."

The Shadow. Tends to hide behind someone more powerful and important. You'll later hear comments about the Shadow like, "Oh! I had no idea Violet was there last night."

The Party Boy. This guy is always dancing with a beer in his hand and mistletoe on his belt buckle (even though it's Memorial Day). He forces off-the-ground bear hugs on everyone who crosses his path, especially Grandma. But don't worry—Grandma likes it!

Mr. Agenda. Has to spray the place with paradoxical statements to show how well he's been doing lately. "It's been a sad year; I had to lay off fifteen of my employees this fall. I felt terrible, but we've gone so hi-tech, I don't really need them anymore," or, "Is it just me, or have you found that supermodels are really lousy in bed?"

The Professor. A true know-it-all. This person loves to amuse his "students" with little-known facts and tidbits about thirteenth-century word origins or the four types of squash served at the first Thanksgiving.

The Topper. This person always has to top the story told. The Topper usually begins a story with "Oh my gosh! You think that's bad?" or "Let me tell *you* about scary . . . !"

The Bar Seeker. When this girl arrives, her number-one mission is to find the bar. She needs a drink, and she needs it fast. And won't talk to anyone until she's had one . . . or six! She's also the person most likely to be found later in the laundry room sleeping on the dryer . . . or your brother!

Meeting my fellow *Celebrity Apprentice* contestants for the first time was the perfect opportunity to observe people entering and reading a room. There's nothing like watching celebrity egos clashing and jockeying for position, especially when officially competing against one another. The guys immediately tried to out–"alpha male" one another. The women spent their first moments sizing up each other's bodies, makeup, and hair, while the guys were checking out our butts. (That first meeting felt like I was at a celebrity dog park!) All the classic party characters were there. We definitely had a Mister Agenda, a Professor, a Party Boy, a couple of Shadows, a few Helpers, more than our share of Swizzle Sticks, and our own Category 5, "Hurricane Omarosa"!

There are times when it is really important to read a room correctly, such as at a job interview, an audition, or even a party or family gathering. As an actress, it's essential to read a room well at auditions, because they make or break your career. Because of this, actors quickly become adept at this kind of interpersonal radar; however, every profession and social situation requires this ability if you want to excel.

The Art of Listening

Listening is at least twice as important as talking. People who have mastered the art of listening are most skilled at reading a room because they have the most perceptive radar. Most people focus on what they're going to say, but what makes a person interesting is how well they listen. Experienced actors have learned to focus not only on saying their lines, but also on listening carefully to the other actors. It is an actor's *reactions* to other actors that make someone interesting in a scene; and it is how you respond to what a person is saying in real life that makes you interesting as a conversationalist. The skill that makes Jay Leno and David Letterman such outstanding talk-show hosts is their acute ability to listen. They are always in present time, and their witty responses come from knee-jerk reactions to what they just heard. They trust themselves to stay with the conversation and allow the punch line to reveal itself based on the last beat, gesture, or comment of the guest.

If you want to really observe how well someone is listening, watch their eyes. The eyes are like a camera, and the camera never lies. The eyes reveal the truth. In fact, the eyes often tell you more than what a person is saying. The first time I went to Italy and stayed with my good friends Maria and Flavio, I spoke no Italian. It was like being a baby again. I would go to parties with all their Italian friends, and without understanding a word at the gathering, I could tell my friends what was going on with each person and how happy or sad or troubled they were. Maria and Flavio would say, "Yes. You're right! How do you know this?" They were always amazed, but I think it's much easier to do this than people realize. The eyes and attitude tell the story. In fact, when you don't have the words to confuse you, you can really tune in to everything else that's going on—the tone, rhythm, eyes, body language, and all the other nonverbal communication.

That particular trip to Italy sharpened my listening skills and my ability to read a room. Taking language out of the equation can help you see what's really going on. Another way to experience this is to watch a foreign movie without subtitles. It is easy to follow what's going on, and you can easily separate the good actors from the bad ones!

Developing communication skills (listening, radar, reading a room, and so on) also comes from having varied social interactions so that you develop the confidence to trust yourself enough to let it flow and be natural. It's very much like studying improvisation as an actor. When you first start classes you want to be really entertaining, so there's a tendency to think ahead while you're in the middle of a scene to try to come up with something funny to say or do. This is exactly what good teachers will tell you *not* to do, because it takes you out of the moment, puts you in your head, and almost always results in boring, canned dialogue and inorganic communication between actors.

After you become more experienced at acting (and especially improv) you learn to trust yourself and *listen* to the other actors and respond in the moment. You basically get out of your head and start "living" on stage rather than "playwriting" in your head. Living and behaving organically are much more compelling to watch for the audience. Playwriting is the kiss of death for everyday social interaction as well, because it's so "studied." I've never been a big fan of actors who seem to be observing themselves from the outside, rather than just behaving. You always get the feeling that they're viewing their performance along with the audience. Worst of all is watching someone on stage stepping all over another actor's lines as though they knew in advance what the actor would say, which of course they do because they've read the script!

Another common mistake is that people sometimes have a certain rhythm in their head of how they *think* a conversation should go. This causes them to force the tone and content of what they're saying, which only makes the conversation feel weird and unnatural. My three-year-old nephew once made a toast at a wedding, saying, "Let's toast to the glasses we hold in our hand." It made no sense, but, to him, he was saying what sounded like the rhythm he heard when grown-ups made toasts in the past. It was actually adorable—because he was three—but adults make this mistake sometimes in conversation. They force a rhythm or interject comments because they're trying to be witty or interesting rather than letting the conversation flow naturally. When I first started doing interviews on television, I would jump into my answer with what I thought was expected of me and based on how it should sound rhythmically, rather than thinking it through and choosing my words based on how I really felt about the question. Don't ever be afraid to take a beat to think about how you really feel about something before answering. You look ridiculous otherwise. (Believe me, I learned the hard way to do this—and in front of millions of people!)

The ability to read a room can be learned from a lot of experience, but it's also inherent in some people. My thirteen-year-old son Nick was born with the ability to read a room. I remember when I was in *Chicago* on Broadway and Nicky had just turned four. In the middle of his good-bye speech to the cast, he said, "And the person I'm really going to miss most is Leigh Zimmerman!" (Leigh is a leggy six-foot-tall dancing goddess Nicky had a big crush on.) As he was saying this, he noticed our best friend in the cast, Michael Berresse, in the crowd, and, to avoid hurting Michael's feelings, Nicky immediately went into an impromptu speech about what a great guy Michael was and how much his friendship meant to us. I couldn't believe I was watching a four-year-old. He took his cue from the reaction he was getting from the audience, and he altered his patter accordingly. Very few people possess the ability to do that at fifty, much less at four. But I do think that lack of radar has less to do with intelligence and more to do with self-consciousness. The more you are focused inward, the less you can focus on what's most important, what's happening around you. It's essential that you are receptive enough to take it all in.

The requirement for reading a room also changes throughout the day and depends on the situation. It is a little more challenging to walk into a group of people already engaged in conversation. You have to be able to sense what's going on to know how, when, and where you should enter, or even *if* you should enter. And then there are other commonplace situations such as greeting friends at work or walking into your home at the end of the day. The greeting or feedback you get from coworkers and family is usually the same. However, every once in a while, there's a difference, and this usually means that something has changed since the last time you were together. The perceptive person is best at finding out what has changed and then knowing what to do about it.

It's also important not to let your emotions get in the way of your radar receptors. Unfortunately, the times when you most need to relax and be your genuine self and keep your radar finely tuned are the times when you're most awkward and anything but your "real" receptive self. Those nerve-wracking times, such as a first date, a job interview, or meeting your new boyfriend's parents or children, can be especially radar-impaired. You'll often hear someone say, "Don't worry, honey, everyone loves you, so just be yourself!" And this *is* good advice. Nothing is more appealing than a person who's natural and comfortable with themselves. When a person is awkward, forcing a personality, or trying to be something they're not, it's so obvious that it makes other people uncomfortable.

Unfortunately, we're least likely to be our comfortable, natural selves when acceptance matters most, and we can say the dumbest, most inappropriate things. I speak from experience when I say that if your ego is prominently hovering over you, and all your focus is turned inward rather than outward, you can entirely miss what's really going on in the room. You become even more self-conscious, which then affects other people, because they pick up on your awkwardness. At that point, they either want to put you out of your misery by taking the conversation away from you, or they start feeling self-conscious, which makes them behave awkwardly, too. The conversation then turns weird, unnatural, and forced, and just goes south from there!

Positive Breeds Positive, Negative Breeds Negative

When performing on Broadway, or on any stage, I always know what kind of performance I'm going to do based on who I know is in the audience. If I know ahead of time, for instance, that my great friend the television mogul Sam Haskell is in the audience, I know I'm going to have a great performance, because Sam is the kind of guy who exudes warmth and confidence. He knows show business extremely well and understands the trial-and-error, hit-or-miss aspect of a performance. When he's watching, I feel as if I'm performing for a proud parent, and I know I can try anything and he'll understand and accept what I'm doing. This freedom usually helps me to have an unselfconscious performance. Being truly open and ready for anything on stage is the most essential ingredient for a great performance. You can miss a step, and yet have access to your instincts enough to know what to do to fix it.

On the other hand, when you know there's someone in the audience who is very critical or judgmental, or has a hovering kind of ego, you can find yourself picking up on their energy. If you're not careful, you can spend your whole performance analyzing yourself as you're saying your lines. You won't be living as the character and staying in the moment. Instead, you'll be living outside yourself, watching your performance like any other spectator. Not to mention that little voice in your head repeating lines and giving negative feedback as you're saying those lines. This is the perfect recipe for a self-conscious, out-of-body performance, which is not fun for an audience to watch.

It's strange that both performances are very similar on the surface, but subtly they are very different, and the audience experiences them on completely different levels. One performance truly moves them emotionally, and the other makes them want to leave early. When people say they felt claustrophobic while watching a performance, it is probably because one of the leads gave a very self-conscious performance, and it rubbed off on the audience.

Audiences don't realize how much they can affect a performance with their feedback. It's a two-way street. If you really want to see a great performance while watching a show, do your best to generate warmth and positive feedback to the performers on stage, and they'll return it in their performance.

Embracing Plan B

Behavior on stage is really not that different from behavior in real life. The more you plan and stay bolted to your agenda, the more difficult it is for people to feel comfortable and natural around you. Part of trusting yourself to stay in the moment is being able to adapt to everything that gets thrown into the mix. How you deal with plan B is one of the most critical aspects of your life.

What do I mean by that? Well, plan A is what we hope will happen or expect to happen, and plan B is often what really happens. I'm also talking about our long-term plans, like what we wanted to be when we grew up, but for now let's just focus on our typical daily plans. Almost every day something turns out different from what we planned. We can either fight it and whine about it or embrace it. I have found that the more I've been open to plan B in life, the more second nature it has become for me. Now I rarely stress about how I want my plans to go. I'm not saying that I don't care. I still plan and care about my plan, but I expect changes and detours to add spice to my expectations.

The best example of this is the way Billy Crystal hosts the Oscars. He writes jokes and prepares for months in advance, yet he comes off as if every joke were spontaneous. This, by the way, is the essence of what makes a great comedian. They always appear spontaneous, even if their material is carefully prepared. I once read that Billy Crystal's joke ratio for the Oscars is something like four or five jokes prepared for every one that actually gets delivered on the show. He's got them all in his back pocket and waits for the perfect opportunity to use them. Most never get used, because the right moment never comes.

My point is that even though this is well planned, the way it actually plays out depends on what actually happens in the moment—the *unplanned* stuff. Billy Crystal is always well prepared for plans B and C and D. Because he's been doing comedy most of his life, he's *always* comfortable with plan B. He could probably do a great job at the Oscars without preparing any jokes at all, but certainly not at the level we've come to expect from him. I think he's the best host in Oscar history.

Embracing plan B is my personal philosophy in life. My first book, an autobiography, was titled *By All Means Keep on Moving*. For me, this means to always forge ahead and make the most of whatever curves life throws you. That is the essence of plan B, whether you're talking about what happened today or your life plans over the last or next twenty years. If you're the type that has to be dragged kicking and screaming into plan B, you're always going to resent having to adjust to what you didn't want. On the other hand, you could try to get excited about the unexpected adventure right around the corner.

If plan B doesn't derail you, but rather inspires you to experience something new, you're allowing yourself to grow with the world around you rather than just the world inside you. I've had so many disappointments in my life, jobs I didn't get, boyfriends who turned out to be jerks, unfaithful, or lazy. Those things always devastated me at first, but most of the time they led to a better job, a better opportunity, and a much better boyfriend. In fact, I'd have to say one of the best jobs of my life, if not *the* best, was *Taxi*, and that was totally a plan B situation. I was set to do another show instead, a one-hour drama. As it turned out, that show got canceled years before *Taxi* ended. So you just never know what's going to happen.

Resilience and Teflon

If I were to choose the most important lesson I want to teach my children, it would have to be to have resilience! The ability to pick yourself up again after a big fall is an ability to be admired. Failure happens to us all, throughout our lives. It's up to you whether you will allow failure to derail you or teach a valuable lesson. What separates winners from losers is the ability to *move on.*

Many people allow themselves to be devastated and derailed when their ego is bruised, instead of using the moment to gain greater insight and perspective on what just happened. A major part of being resilient is in knowing yourself. When you have confidence and know who you are as a person, what others say about you doesn't affect you in the way it affects someone who lacks that confidence and self-awareness. If anything, the confident person welcomes the opportunity to get another perspective and greater insight from the criticism. Chances are when you hear something negative about yourself, it's not the first time you've heard it; there's often at least *some* truth to it. People tend to get offended mostly by the criticisms that they believe are true and valid. I never get offended by comments that I don't believe in my heart to be true. I naturally discount them as the opinion of someone who is not very well informed or who lacks understanding or experience to make a judgment that I respect enough to take seriously.

Resilience is just as important a component in communication as radar and your ability to read a room. You need to develop the ability to coat yourself with Teflon—metaphorically, of course. I always use Teflon to mean that little coat of protection you need to shield yourself from the slings and arrows of others. There are so many times when everything is going great in a social situation, you're reading the room perfectly, and your receptors are working at full capacity, and then someone makes a comment that offends you or bruises your ego so much that you can no longer objectively focus on what's happening. All you can do is ruminate over what that person just said. You are then no longer in present time and no longer in sync with what's happening. The people who seem to get injured the most are those who accept a comment or criticism as a narcissistic injury. They take it so personally that they can't recover from it, rather than understanding the why behind it.

In short, when your attention units are tuned outward, you can take in and appreciate your surroundings—what you're observing in other people and your environment. But when your attention units are focused inward, you're full of stress and self-consciousness, which is uninteresting to watch and uncomfortable to be around. The next time you are in a social situation, allow yourself to simply listen for fifteen minutes. Don't put any pressure on yourself to interject. Feel free to say something if you are compelled to, but don't feel any *need* to speak. The point is to *really* focus on listening. What usually happens is that you automatically respond in a pertinent manner because you become truly engaged in what's happening.

> *I still have a vision in my mind [from] the first time I encountered the idea of Teflon in a class. In my mind I saw all of us in class lined up and getting this showering coat of Teflon over our well-selected outfits. It made us feel protected and allowed us to explore and tackle new ideas and challenges without fear. Our own little superhero suit.*
>
> —DORIS PENDERGRASS,
> Maryland,
> Marilu.com member

> *As a former approval junkie, the idea of Teflon has made a big difference in my happiness and peace of mind. A small dose of indifference to what people think of me at any given moment frees me up to be true to myself and be the BEST person I can be.*
>
> —CATHY DODD,
> Washington,
> Marilu.com member

Wrapping It Up!

- You can't develop a strong personality at home alone in your basement.

- Listening is at least twice as important as talking.

- If you want to really observe how well someone is listening, watch their eyes.

- Taking language out of the equation can help you see what's really going on.

- Don't let your emotions get in the way of your radar receptors.

- Will failure derail you or teach a valuable lesson? It's your choice.

- The confident person welcomes the opportunity to get another perspective and greater insight from criticism.

Seven

USE IT OR LOSE IT

"I'm so tired!"

"I can't remember anything!"

"I can't move like I used to."

"I'd like to go back to college, but I can't handle the workload . . . or brain load!"

I've heard complaints like these many times. These are the typical fears people start to have in their thirties and forties. What often leads to this kind of thinking is that we stop doing something we did regularly, such as exercising, taking classes, or working outside the home, and when we make an attempt to go back, it seems more challenging than ever before. We become discouraged and question our abilities. One of three things usually happens then: One, we postpone our attempts long enough and never bother trying. Two, we make a genuine attempt to go back, but find ourselves too overwhelmed to continue on that path. Or three, we actually stay with it long enough to truly adapt and eventually realize that it wasn't age holding us back at all, but rather lack of conditioning and genuine commitment.

The expression "use it or lose it" is most often used to kid older people about their sex lives, and, even though it's meant as a tease, it's great advice! Studies show that regular sex is one of the best ways to preserve your sexual prowess. Unfortunately, there is a tendency for people to hold back at times (or at least use that as an excuse) in order to conserve their energy and resources so they'll be ready to go when needed. Nothing could be further from the truth! Our bodies and minds don't work like a car or a toaster oven. Those items wear down and eventually need to be replaced. With humans, and all animals for that matter, the *more* you do, the more you *can* do and want to do! Tiger Woods would never take it easy a month or two before a major. He, like every athlete, needs to train regularly before every competition in order to condition his body and mind to handle the intensity of the competition. And that's golf! Imagine the preparation for an Olympic marathon or the Tour de France.

Use it or lose it is not only true for sports and sex. Nearly everything we do in life is based on this principle. It goes down to our basic cellular level. Take vaccinations, for example. A low or inactive dose of a disease is injected into your body to stimulate your immune system to produce antibodies against that disease. In a sense it gives your body a chance to practice a little war against the disease so it will be ready to take on the real disease if it attacks. It's your body's own Army Reserve system. Native Americans suffered a population catastrophe in the sixteenth century when a high percentage of them died, primarily because their immune systems had no experience dealing with smallpox and other European diseases. Everybody and everything in life—including the tiniest cells in your body—needs experience and practice. It should be no surprise that our skills increase when we are challenged in that area.

Use Your Brain!

Perhaps the most important category of *use it or lose it* is the function of the brain. The latest research on this has been very encouraging. It turns out that cognitive problems and memory loss are not normal. They may be relatively common, but they are certainly not normal or necessary. Research shows that people experience memory loss more often from *understimulation* than from what most people assume to be the natural aging process. There is no reason to "expect" memory loss as you get older. The brain is much more adaptable and capable of growth than formerly thought. New neurons are formed after physical and mental activity, even in older adults. (Very reassuring for us baby boomers!)

The human brain is so powerful, and yet we habitually use just a small percentage of its potential. If we get in the habit of using it more and more each day, our brain capacity can grow exponentially.

But you've got to *use your brain*!

I say this to my kids at least once a day, along with my mom's favorite, "If you're bored, you're boring!" Too often we avoid using our brains out of sheer laziness, but many of us don't use our brains out of simple habit. Think about it. Every time we use speed dial or spell-check, write things down instead of memorizing them, or access one of our online "favorites," we're missing an opportunity for daily brain exercise. Just the way you might park far away from your destination to get in that extra workout or take the stairs instead of an elevator, grab daily opportunities to exercise your brain!

For example, don't use speed dial unless it's absolutely necessary. Instead of writing down information, commit it to memory by using word and visual association techniques. Listen to lectures on tape instead of music in your car. And if you really want to use your brain, before you go grocery shopping, write out a list aisle by aisle, based on your memory of the store's layout. Don't even look at the list as you're shopping, but see if you can remember everything in order on your list. Check it just before you leave the store to see how well you did. I play this little game often, and because of it, I rarely even need a list anymore. Finally, before you put anything in your mouth today, use your brain to determine if you really should be eating it. Remember, a strong brain equals strong willpower!

Use Your Body

Obviously it is very important to exercise both your brain *and* body regularly, because diseases of the body negatively affect the brain and vice versa. Many people focus on one and not the other, but exercising *both* is essential! It's common to see people who can't tear themselves away from their books but haven't worn a pair of sneakers in years, and equally common to see Barbie and Ken types jumping and pumping iron two or three hours a day but not exercising their brains through reading or study.

In addition to this, a reduction in *social* interaction can have a negative effect on your mental and emotional well-being. A study by Duke University's Center for the Study of Aging and Human Development stated, "Retirement had the most negative social-psychological effects. . . . Early retirement may reduce communication and thinking skills." When stand-up or improv comedians return to performing after a long hiatus, they need to exercise their "funny bones" to get back to the mindset, speed, and timing that are required to perform well. This is similar to how most people feel when they haven't been socially interactive for a while. It can be very intimidating for a person to return to the dating scene after a divorce or the death of a spouse—even flirting is a "muscle" that needs to be exercised!

Physical inactivity is the most obvious example of use it or lose it. When a person wears a cast for a month or more, the lack of muscle stimulation causes noticeable muscle atrophy by the time the cast is removed. The book *The Raft* is a true account of three strong, young Air Force pilots in World War II who were stranded for twenty-eight days on a small rubber raft in the Pacific Ocean. When rescued, they were unable to walk or even stand up after just four weeks of inactivity and very limited amounts of protein. They suffered severe atrophy. When astronauts are in space for even a few days, they routinely do resistance training on the spacecraft in order to prevent atrophy.

My Exercise Routine

I love exercise. I know that sounds a little strange to some people, but exercise brings me immeasurable joy! It's one of my true passions in life. Some people hate even hearing the word *exercise*, much less doing it, but I've never felt that way. If I don't do some form of exercise every day, even if it's just walking around my neighborhood, then I don't feel like *me*.

The benefits of exercise are endless. It reduces stress, lowers blood pressure and cholesterol, controls weight, burns fat, combats osteoporosis, builds, strengthens, and tones muscles, slows the aging process, balances your mood, and makes you feel great, too! Yet, incredibly, 80 percent of Americans don't do it regularly (defined as more than twice a week). I used to be baffled by this. I could not comprehend why so many people would avoid doing something that is so great for you and makes you feel so good. But I now understand the reason for this paradox. Most people associate exercise with going to the gym three or more times a week, pumping iron, doing high-impact aerobics or step class, and sweating over a spin bike. For some people and personality types, this is the perfect environment for breaking a sweat. Some people thrive in a gym, and that's great! They should continue to enjoy what's working for them. But for many—perhaps the 80 percent who are *not* exercising—this may be the wrong prescription for fitness. They need to find an alternative that inspires them.

The most essential ingredient for long-term success is that it *must* be something you enjoy doing! If you don't enjoy doing it, you won't continue doing it. It's that simple. Whatever you choose to do must be something you look forward to doing three, four, or even more times a week. You may think it's impossible for you to feel that way about exercise, especially if you *hate* exercise, but I believe that people who don't enjoy exercising are those who haven't yet found the exercise that suits them best. They haven't found their exercise "soul mate"! They haven't found the body movement that brings them joy. Deriving bliss from movement is natural for *everyone* who is part of the animal kingdom. Think about it. Animals love to and need to *move*. As I'm always telling people who are exercise haters, "You walk your dog, your cat stretches, and your hamster gets on that wheel. You are this beautiful human animal, so get off your butt and move your body!"

Perhaps this reluctance to exercise stems from the misconception that it has to follow some strict guidelines of lifting, training, and straining, and that the more fun movements like ballroom dancing, tennis, badminton, and golf are just part of playtime. But studies show that, although these more enjoyable activities may not condition your body as efficiently as the Jack LaLanne or the pumping iron–type exercises, they are still quite beneficial for your fitness, health, energy, and especially your well-being.

Movement in itself is beneficial. Movement *is* exercise! Don't ever feel like you're not exercising because you're having too much fun. That's exactly the point. It *has* to be fun. Most important, it has to be something you will actually do! I don't care how efficient your workouts are; if you do them only six times a year, they're worthless. So first find the exercises you enjoy doing. Get moving first, and then, if you get more ambitious later, add the barbells. You need to first find your exercise "soul mate"!

Mine for the last twenty-eight years has been Pilates. I occasionally take a short break from Pilates. I might even have a summer fling with yoga or flamenco. But, amazingly, after all these years, I'm still in the honeymoon phase with Pilates.

I first took a Pilates class on January 4, 1979. It seemed different from all the dancing exercises I'd been doing since I was five years old, but I felt instantly connected to it. I love moving in positions that specifically target one spot, yet, strangely enough, these moves engage my whole body. I love the idea of fluid motion. Pilates is not as static as yoga. It constantly moves. I see it as a combination of dance and yoga, and it has taught me how to breathe more efficiently and to become more aware of proper body alignment. I found Pilates during the Jane Fonda workout era and, as much as I loved blasting music and doing aerobics, Pilates felt more grounded and nurturing for my body. Perhaps what I love most about it is that I feel energized after class rather than exhausted, and I always leave class with a greater body awareness and better posture, which stay with me the rest of the day. And that body awareness gets recharged every time I take a class.

Now, what if you haven't yet found your exercise soul mate—or mates? How do you begin your search? This, in my opinion, is the most exciting part of the process. It's kind of like dating and playing the field! Spend an hour or so online, making calls, gathering brochures, and so on. This is the "speed dating" phase to help you choose with whom you want to "go out." Explore YMCAs, community colleges, health clubs, boxing clubs, karate schools, and dance studios. Don't limit yourself; consider everything and then start taking trial classes. If you don't like a class, don't do it again! If you like it, try a second class "date." If you think you may have found a love connection, sign up for a whole semester. If you want to save money, go to the library and check out a new exercise or dance video every week. You can spend the rest of your life in this phase, trying new things. It's not as if you have to find just one thing and stay monogamous. Don't be afraid to be an exercise hussy! In fact, variety is the best thing for your body, not just targeting one group of sports-specific muscles. It's good to work your entire body over the whole range of motion.

I always find it helpful to work from a list, so here are some suggestions to help spark ideas: tennis, golf, swimming, racquetball, tai chi, tap dancing, ballet, jazz, modern, flamenco, ballroom (swing, Latin, waltz, tango), karate, judo, aerobics, skiing, skating, rowing, diving, jogging, walking, ping-pong, badminton, and basketball.

Everybody has a different exercise personality; perhaps classes or team sports aren't for you. Some people thrive when they can compete against themselves or a friend. Consider taking the President's Fitness Challenge. This is a way to shoot for a specific fitness goal. The President's Challenge is a program that has been around since Kennedy was in office. It encourages all age groups to make fitness a part of their everyday lives. No matter what your activity and fitness level, the President's Challenge can help motivate you to improve. This is a fun way to start a challenging fitness program with your family and friends. Go to www.presidentschallenge.org for more information and to sign up.

Taking Action

Once you make some choices, it's time to get down to business. It's sometimes difficult for people to take action, but once they get into a class, on a court, or in the field and start moving, they're fine. That's why it's important to make exercise as convenient as possible. It's easier to exercise when all your stuff is organized and ready to go. Your first task is to gather *everything* you own that has something to do with your workouts: sweats, sneakers, shorts, balls, bats, racquets, caps, T-shirts, iPod, fanny packs, dumbbells, and resistance bands. You're basically taking exercise inventory.

Don't think of your exercise clothing as the oldest, most beat-up T-shirts, sweats, or shorts you own. Choose workout clothes that are comfortable both physically *and* emotionally. Make it easy on the eyes as well as the mind. It's difficult to work out when you feel self-conscious. Wear outfits that show off your best assets in class or at the gym and that will inspire you to work out harder, longer, and with more focus. Always choose workout clothes that breathe well, too. Go with 100 percent cottons over synthetic blends. Polyester and vinyl delude people into thinking they're losing more weight because of increased perspiration. This water loss is only temporary, and you tend to work out much less when you are overheated and uncomfortable. Vinyl sweats can, in fact, be dangerous because they cause dehydration.

Research shows that only one in three people who have home exercise equipment (such as free weights, treadmills, and Stairmasters) use it regularly. This is probably partly because the home environment is much less stimulating than a gym, which has lots of people, bright lights, loud music, and perhaps some competition. My brother Lorin always says he can do thirty-five push-ups alone and fifty if a girl is watching. If you work out at home, create tricks to motivate yourself, such as blasting invigorating music and dancing around the house.

Once you've gathered everything you've got, designate one specific spot (dresser drawer, box, barrel, chest, or trunk) to situate all exercise gear and equipment. Choose a spot that's highly accessible and easy to keep clean and organized. Consider a full-length mirror as part of your workout gear and place it close to where you work out. I believe a mirror can sometimes be a better fitness tool than a scale, because it helps you check your alignment and adjust your posture while it keeps you focused on your goals and inspires energy surges throughout your workout. If you find the opposite to be true, however, then by all means hide the mirror until you're ready for it . . . if ever! Do whatever is necessary for success.

Another good idea is to keep some exercise equipment and workout clothes in the trunk of your car. You never know when you'll have the opportunity for a good workout. Many times I find myself walking around the block instead of sitting in a waiting room because I've kept supplies on hand. Always be ready if the time or mood presents itself. Once that moment passes, it's difficult to get it back.

And here's one last exercise suggestion for those of you who are too busy to exercise: Design your own simple twenty-minute workout, and then break it down into four five-minute workouts that can be done anywhere, anytime. I've found that the best movements for this are exercises like leg lifts, calf raises, sit-ups, deep knee bends, and pliés. And don't be afraid to use resistance bands or light dumbbells. Think simple, light, and low injury risk. Then incorporate those four mini-workouts somewhere in your busy day: at the bus stops, next to the copy machine, in front of the television, or while waiting for dinner to cook.

One last thought about exercise: Maintaining a regular exercise regimen is not only important to preserve and improve muscle tone; it is equally important to maintain healthy bones and delay the onset of osteoporosis. Strength-training exercises (free weights, weight machines, and resistance bands) and weight-bearing semi-aerobic exercises (walking, jazz and ballet dancing, low-impact aerobics, and step classes) strengthen the muscles and bones in your arms, legs, torso, and upper spine and also work directly on your bones to slow mineral loss.

Keep in mind that abrupt, straining, jerky movements are harmful to your body. Sports such as soccer, rugby, racquetball, and tennis are more likely than other sports to cause injuries, so it's important to use caution and do those activities in moderation, especially in your thirties and older. Overtraining of any kind or training without properly warming up and stretching is always risky. Too much of anything or the wrong kind of exercise is dangerous. Don't confuse "use it or lose it" with *over*use it!

I knew I loved exercise (especially Pilates), but I never realized just how important it was to me until recently when, for two weeks, I was unable to do it. Absence *does* make the heart grow fonder. I know it sounds crazy, but that was the longest I'd ever gone without exercising since I was a teenager. I craved it. I missed it. I couldn't stand it. When I don't exercise I don't feel at my best. Perhaps it's because I was so active as a child. I started dancing when I was very young, and I was always a bit of a tomboy (even though I play sports like a girly girl). I'm more like a tom*girl*. I take big strides when I walk, and I just never stop moving. My father's nickname for me as a kid was Perpetual Motion. I liked that name so much, it's now the name of my corporation. My son Nicky said to me, "When I think of you, Mom, I always think of you moving." That was such a compliment to me because it confirmed my father's nickname and persona for me when I was even younger than Nicky. It was almost as if my father were speaking to me through my son.

Exercise to me is like brushing your teeth or even breathing. It's not just something I like to do every day; it's something I *need* to do every day. Without exercise I feel as if my brain doesn't function as it should and my digestive tract doesn't work properly. Our whole body "factory" begins to malfunction when we go without exercise. A sad statistic that illustrates this is that the average life expectancy after a person breaks their hip is only fifteen years. I'm sure a lot of that stems from a significant reduction of mobility. In extreme cases of inactivity, such as severe paralysis, the life expectancy is less than ten years.

Deriving bliss from movement is natural for *everyone* who is part of the animal kingdom. Whether it's that hamster on a wheel, neurons in your brain, cells in your immune system, or lions and wildebeests on the Serengeti, all living things, especially us (*especially* wilde-beests!), need to use it or they'll lose it!

Wrapping It Up!

- The *more* you do, the more you *can* do and *want* to do!

- *Use it or lose it* is not only true for sports and sex. Everything we do is based on this principle, down to our basic cellular level.

- There is no reason to "expect" memory loss as you get older. The brain is much more adaptable and capable of growth than formerly thought.

- Get in the habit of using your brain more each day, and its capacity can grow exponentially.

- It's very important to exercise both your brain *and* body.

- A reduction in social interaction can have a negative effect on your mental and emotional well-being.

- Exercise reduces stress, lowers blood pressure and cholesterol, controls weight, burns fat, combats osteoporosis, builds, strengthens, and tones muscles, slows the aging process, balances your mood, and makes you feel great!

- The most essential ingredient for long-term success is that the exercise you choose must be something you enjoy doing.

- Make exercise as convenient as possible.

- Our whole body "factory" begins to malfunction when we go without exercise.

Eight

SHARPEN YOUR PRESENTATION

When I refer to presentation, I'm talking about the whole package of how you are perceived, which includes your appearance, persona, communication skills, idiosyncrasies, and everything else that communicates to the world who you are. All of these are important. In fact, they are much more important than we want to admit as a society. Like it or not, people *do* judge a book, and people, by its cover, and that's why it's essential to devote a lot of energy to developing a great cover—your presentation!

Communication Skills

I have known many people over the years who were loaded with talent, but because they were intimidated about speaking in public, they never developed strong communication skills. They are very funny or insightful, but put them anywhere near someone unfamiliar, or worse, in front of a crowd, and their entire personality disappears! Unfortunately, this inability to be who they are or get their message across usually prevents them from reaching their full potential in their careers and relationships. Strong public-speaking skills, along with the talent to communicate personably and effectively, can reap immeasurable benefits throughout your profession and in your personal life. For this reason, I've always encouraged my kids to get involved in projects that develop social skills after school and in the summer. Fortunately, they are now fearless when it comes to meeting new people, playing sports, or getting up on stage in front of adults or peers. (Sometimes a little too fearless!)

I know that one of the strongest assets to my career as an actress has been that I've never shied away from being on talk shows. My one-thousand-plus talk-show appearances fortified my career from the beginning because they kept me frequently in the public eye and helped support and sell whatever project I was working on. It also doesn't hurt that, because every appearance is potentially seen by hundreds of prominent agents and casting directors, I have gotten many jobs because someone saw me on *The Tonight Show*! Many professional actors, however, miss golden opportunities to do press for their latest projects because they're afraid of being themselves on talk shows. And these are actors! They are *used* to appearing in front of people. Imagine how difficult it is for many businessmen to present a monthly report in the boardroom, or for a young attorney to present her first case in court. Some actors I know have even quit the business because they had so much anxiety about doing interviews and talk shows.

People often ask me what it takes to be a good guest on a talk show, and I always say, "It's exactly the same as what makes someone interesting in everyday life or at a party. You have to ride the wave of a conversation. You have to be in present time by taking in what's going on in the moment, and making sure that what you contribute is real and heartfelt." How you are truly feeling about something in the moment—being really connected in mind, heart, and words—is always compelling to other people. You can even memorize the bullet points of your own agenda, but if you're too fixed on telling a long, detailed story, or on something you had planned to say, it will not only come off robotic and stiff and boring, it will also feel disconnected to the reality of what's happening at that very moment. I'll never forget seeing Sharon Stone on Letterman when she took a piece of paper from her shoe and proceeded to read her own Top Ten list. It was out of sync with what was happening on the show at that moment. The way she did it showed that she obviously pictured the whole scene in her head beforehand, but it played out differently on the show, and instead of adjusting and reacting to what Dave and the audience were doing, she continued with her own agenda. After she left, Dave said, "Is it my imagination, or did everything we talk about end in a cul-de-sac?" She may be a beautiful woman and actress, but she is very strange on talk shows.

You can tell which people are "there" in present time. I once had an acting teacher who could watch someone's performance, and he could always tell the difference between the people who were in the moment from those who had practiced in front of a mirror. When a "practiced" actor, with his telltale glazed look, finished a scene, the teacher would say, "You were in the land where elephants die." And he was right! The actor looked a million miles away. It didn't matter if he was at home in front of a mirror or in front of an audience; his performance would have looked the same, because it had nothing to do with where he was or with whom he was performing. I can't overemphasize the importance of staying in the moment. It's the difference between being fresh or stale. Don't, however, confuse being in the moment with not doing your homework or being well prepared for the speech you are delivering or the subject you will be discussing.

Expert Advice

I often feature guest lecturers in my classes at Marilu.com, and one of the most compelling and inspirational speakers is Tom Alderman, president and founder of MediaPrep Inc. Tom has trained hundreds of celebrities, executives, authors, and teachers how to communicate most effectively. He always says that when giving a speech, making a presentation, or interviewing for a job, the first thing you have to understand is that it's not only about the content you're conveying; it's also about the performance you're giving. You can't separate the two. He often cites the research out of Stanford University that found that 93 percent of what an audience gets from your message is based on you—your demeanor, delivery, and attitude—which leaves only 7 *percent* for the carefully crafted words that you used. Image is almost everything—scary but true. No wonder we're a little self-conscious when getting up in front of a crowd. We should be! In the words of an old Fats Waller song that Alderman cites, "It ain't what you say, it's the way that you say it."

As Alderman also says, "Content without demeanor is like a hook without the bait." In any act of communication, whether it's one-on-one, for a small group, or for a million TV viewers, you're always in performance mode. The stakes are even higher if you're really trying to get a point across or impress somebody. You click into a performance mode that says to the other person, "There's no other place I want to be right now than here talking to you." Alderman also explained that it's not unlike talking to your spouse or children. When parents are angry and lose their temper, their child may not fully understand why they're mad, but they'll definitely *feel* the anger. That feeling is what carries the message.

Eye contact with your audience is crucial, but it's important not to stare. Some people don't like direct eye contact, and others are uncomfortable with close proximity. This is one of the reasons it's so important to focus on your demeanor—the 93 percent. Be aware of *how* you're relaying your message along with the content of *what* you are saying. I've met people who could say "Pass the salt" and it sounds like they're swearing at you, and then there are people who are actually using profanity and it sounds like a nursery rhyme. Psychologists, for example, are more interested in a person's body language and affect than what the person is actually saying.

A simple "Hi" from a business colleague can ruin your day or brighten your spirits depending on the attitude behind it. A cheerful "Hi" says "I'm happy to see you," and a grumpy "Hi" says "Don't bother me now!" When you really want to communicate, you *must* be an active listener, being in the moment and continually playing back what others are saying to you. If you are at a job interview, it's important to stay thoroughly engaged in the conversation, but also sit forward in your chair so that your physical message aligns with your actual engagement. Never slouch; it diminishes your energy and implies to your companion that you might have a better place to be than where you are at that moment. It is no accident that the set of *Larry King Live* is around a table, because it forces people to shift forward when they talk, as they should at a job interview.

Now what about that other 7 percent—the control over your words and the message you want to get across? Alderman teaches that whenever you walk into a meeting with an employer or employee, you have to decide ahead of time the one, two, or three core messages that you want to get across. Research out of UCLA demonstrates that an audience can retain up to, but not more than, three core messages.

Three is fine, but it's better to narrow it to two. Let's say, for example, the two messages for your job interview are that you are superior in your field and you know how to get the job done by working well with a team. Don't be afraid to subtly send those messages several times throughout your conversation in the way you answer your interview questions. Repetition is a strong way to get your message across as long as you don't overdo it.

One last thing about job interviews: When Ben Franklin was asked the appropriate attire for Congress, he said, "Wear a benign smile. A benign smile carries the day."

What about a situation in which you have to reprimand an employee for lateness or less-than-stellar performance? Alderman suggests two tacks: First, decide the one, two, or three points you want to make, but use a supportive demeanor so that you don't put the person on the defensive. Second, simply listen to the person's problems and concerns; ask a lot of questions pertaining to how they're feeling and what they're feeling. This strategy may not always work with a disgruntled employee, but at least you are doing your part to create the most favorable environment for open communication. Professionals also use an important word-control method called the alignment technique: If the person interviewing you expresses a concern or a problem, first align yourself with the concern before you try to change the person's opinion. The only way you're going to sway someone's opinion is to first demonstrate that you understand *their* position. People rarely do this with coworkers, family members, or spouses. This tack can completely change the outcome of most arguments. Frequently this softens both sides and a common ground is reached quickly.

Tom Alderman's information was so helpful to the members of Marilu.com that one of the women took his advice the following day at an interview and landed the job of a lifetime!

It's All about Homework

As much as I always emphasize being in the moment and trusting yourself enough to "let it flow," the key to this is being so prepared that you naturally have the confidence to allow yourself to be in present time. That's why I am a strong believer in doing your homework.

When the producers first called me about doing *Chicago* on Broadway, I had been getting a little exercise raising my boys, but I wasn't anywhere near the shape I needed to be in to star in a Broadway musical—a Bob Fosse musical, no less! I was more in mommy mode than *Mama Mia!* mode. They were considering me to replace Ann Reinking, the legendary Fosse dancer (as well as Bob's ex-girlfriend) who originated the Roxie role in the *Chicago* revival. They asked how much dancing I'd been doing lately, and I deftly changed the subject. The truth was that I hadn't had my legs up in the air since the night I gave birth . . . and the time before that was the night I got pregnant!

I needed to get my butt back to class ASAP, so I called my brother Lorin, my former dancing buddy and cohort on my exercise video *Dancerobics*. Neither of us had been in a dance class in years, but we did our best to dust off our Boogie Fever jazz pants and character shoes and chasséd off to the nearest dance studio in Hollywood. (Denny Terrio would have been proud!) The class was physically and emotionally traumatic for both of us, and even worse for the people in the observation room! At one point I saw poor Lorin grimacing at his wristwatch while struggling through a long set of pas de chats. *Pas de chat* is a French ballet term meaning "step of the cat." I was feeling like a cat all right, but it was Grizabella, the grungy flea magnet who sings "Memory" in *Cats*.

I could actually hear the sounds of creaking bones and rusty cartilage. They were saying, "Oooiiilll. Ooooiiiilll!" Lorin turned to me at the end of the class and said, "When word gets out, there's going to be a recall on *Dancerobics!*"

As bad as we were, I was not discouraged. Driving home, all I could think about was how much I wanted this part and that I was going to do everything in my power to make it happen. I officially embraced the challenge! (Cue the theme from *Rocky*.)

I had exactly one week to get in shape before flying to New York for my audition, so I started bright and early the next morning and took every jazz and ballet class I could sink my feet into before my flight. I got my dancer legs on faster than I thought, but I still had no idea what I was getting myself into.

When I arrived, the first thing I did was see the show. Afterward I was struck with two thoughts. One, "I have to get this part!" And two, "Oh my gosh! How am I ever going to get my body to contort in that unique, incredibly sexy Fosse way?" Most of his movements and positions are not what your body naturally wants to do, but it is mandatory to do them if you want that look, even though your muscles have to stretch a specific way first.

The next morning I went to the first audition. I didn't know it at the time, but I was dressed completely wrong. I felt confident, but I had no right to be. They were seeing only two Roxies that day, and the other one was Sandahl Bergman, an old friend who had been the lead dancer in the Fosse biography *All That Jazz*. It's a little like trying out for *Funny Girl* and having Barbra Streisand walk in.

Sandahl was amazing. She instantly picked up the routine after seeing it just once. Her body positions and movements were the epitome of the Fosse style. Instead of competing with her, I tried my best to copy her. (It felt like I was cheating on a midterm!) We did our dancing audition together, but they separated us for our singing and acting auditions, which I felt went well. Before I left, they told me that although they weren't ready to make a decision just yet, I should go back to Los Angeles, really practice, keep dancing, and *especially* work on absorbing the Fosse technique into my body.

I left with the feeling that I scored well in every category but Fosse, so *that's* what I focused on. I beelined it to the video store to stock up on Fosse films. As soon as I started watching *All That Jazz* I recognized a dancer friend, Kathryn Doby, whom I called immediately and asked to be my Fosse tutor. She told me she was leaving for Hungary on Monday but that we had the weekend to blitz on Bob. The soundtrack in my head changed to *Eye of the Tiger*, followed by a montage sequence with Kathryn showing me lots of hand positions, hip isolations, back arches, hat poses, and a sexy Fosse fashion show with high heels, sheer black hose, and leg-extending French-cut leotards. (The song slowly fades out as we giggle through an eye makeup workshop, a la *Laverne and Shirley*.)

By the time the Marilu movie fantasy ended in my head, I found myself back in New York for my second audition facing a room full of Broadway all-stars. Everyone I idolized in show business was there on both sides of the desk. Instead of being intimidated, I couldn't wait to strut my stuff. *I aced it!* I was there for a grueling three-and-a-half hours, but nothing threw me because *I was prepared*! I knew by the end of the work session that I had the job.

Now, I don't want to give the impression that all I needed to get the part was two weeks of intensive training. Those two weeks were in addition to the twenty-five years of show-business experience that I had already brought to the table, including a lot of homework-cramming weekends for past auditions whenever I felt shorthanded in one particular aspect, as I did this time with the Fosse technique. What's important is identifying your shortcomings and then doing your homework to compensate for them. There's nothing like being prepared for anything that's thrown at you. It is, by far, one of the greatest feelings in life!

Detox Your Style

Now let's talk about the outer cover of your presentation—your appearance and style. Going back to the Fats Waller song, I need to add that it ain't *just* what you say or how you say it; it's also about how you *look* when you're saying it. Like it or not, appearance and style matter big time. It's important to be in charge of your own personal style.

To begin with, do you actually *have* a personal style? Your personal style is important because it tells people who you are, what you want, and what people should expect of you. Does your style match up with what you want your image to be? When people look at you, what's the first thing they see? What kind of statement are you making? Do people see you as someone who settles for whatever was available in your closet that morning? Or are you seen as someone who makes an effort? Are you perhaps a work in progress or a blank slate?

Starting out as an actress, for a long time my style was just a blank slate. I didn't really know who I was, and I tried on many looks and styles that were wrong. I was kind of like "eclectic" Barbie, but I wanted to be "Marilu" Barbie (similar to Malibu Barbie, but without the surfboard). I was so happy when I finally found a look that felt like *me*! I realized after much trial and error what colors, styles, and lines worked with my body and made me feel like I was wearing the clothes rather than they were wearing me. (Another example of wear your life well!) It felt great because it helped me define my persona as an actress. Once people are clear about who you are (because the outer and inner you are connected), they know how to place you and cast you. This is true not only for actors but for every career. If you act like the manager and present yourself like a manager, eventually people will make you the manager. If you act like the lowly errand boy, you'll stay the lowly errand boy.

I always feel that a good place to start when developing your personal style is at the top—*your hair*. Your hair makes or breaks your look. I always say that hair is the "B Story" because no matter what the main event of the day is, hair always plays a prominent supporting role. It's a major part of the big picture and usually the first thing people notice about you, even before your smile, because it frames your face and shapes your silhouette. You never hear somebody saying, "I had a bad makeup day" or "I had a bad wardrobe day." It's only "a bad hair day." Ask yourself, "How long have I had this look?" A common problem with hair is that people find a style that works for them, and then they lock it in for . . . *decades*! They don't want to mess with success, so they try to preserve their high school look all the way to the nursing home. Are you possibly wearing the same hairstyle you had in high school or college?

People tend to make their best effort in high school and college; it's the time when women experiment most with hair and makeup. After that, many people don't change their hairstyle until it thins out or goes gray—if then! You can often tell what year someone graduated by their hairstyle.

If you first learned hairstyling using hot rollers or pin curls, a straightening iron, Velcro rollers, or a crimping iron, there's a good chance you're still using them now. What about your hair products? Have they changed over the years? Are you still using Dippity Doo from the 1970s, mousse from the 1980s, styling lotion and gels from the 1990s, creams from the early 2000s? Some styles mark an era because so many people copy a popular celebrity look and that style becomes almost unavoidable (think Jennifer Aniston or Farrah Fawcett). You may think, "Gosh! I really want Beyonce's hair," but instead of wearing her exact style, it's much wiser to choose a style that works for *you*.

I've noticed similarities with makeup. What look was popular when you started wearing makeup, and how much has your look evolved since then? A high school girl will learn her makeup technique based on current trends, and then it becomes like paint-by-number. It's important to experiment and break the mold if you're stuck in a makeup rut. This is true even for professionals. I can often tell in which era makeup artists started in the business because they tend to use the same products and techniques that were popular when they joined the union.

This is true not only for hair and makeup but also for many other aspects of our lives. People tend to do the same dance steps they learned in their teens and twenties. If you go to a dance attended by seniors in their seventies and eighties, you'll see them doing the same steps they did in high school and college. People my age are still most comfortable doing disco. It's almost as if people define their lives based on who they were in their late teens, and they rarely experiment with styles and trends that follow. Those things, unfortunately, become less important as we get older, but they shouldn't. Change is fun, and experimenting with your style makes you more exciting as a person.

Now, I'm not suggesting that we all wear micro mini skirts, expose our midriffs, and pierce our navels, but it can be very exciting to play with newer clothing and hairstyles that are appropriate for who you are and who you want to be. And please go ahead and learn some fun new dance steps and even pass them on to your *elders*. (Don't you wish your grandma was *hot* like me? And how cool would she look doing Soulja Boy!)

The best way to develop a style is through observation and trial and error. Whenever you find a look that doesn't work for you, analyze why. Often it's a fitness or weight issue, but after you lose a few or hit the gym, a style that didn't work before looks very flattering. Aside from helping you feel great and be healthier, a program of eating right and exercising regularly also gives you the benefit of looking good in a wider range of styles. Even cheaper clothes can look like a million bucks, so getting fit and healthy is a money saver, too!

It's also fun to experiment with color. What's the first color you grab when you see a rack of clothes? For me it's always been black, but I now realize that navy and chocolate brown are my BFFs (best friends forever)! They simply look better with my skin tone and hair color. Clothes with color look better on camera, too, so keep that in mind when having your picture taken. Black clothes in photos or on TV create a vacuum image, almost a "black hole," but navy or brown adds warmth and a definable shape while still giving you a nice, dark (and slimming!) silhouette.

Along with experimenting with color, learn to observe what you see in magazines, on the street, and in clothing stores, and pay attention to how people dress on TV. Go shopping with a friend who has a lot of style to get her fresh perspective and a second opinion. Let her pick out things that are different from what you would normally pick, and try to see yourself through her eyes.

It's also very important to get familiar with your body type. Once you really understand your shape, you will have a much easier time finding the clothes that complement you most. If you get really perceptive at this, you can also find which designer's clothes work best for your body type and shape. Each designer works with a fit model, or models, and they develop their styles based on the models they work with. If you are similarly shaped to their fit model(s), their clothes will fit like they were made for you. There are certain designers and brands I cannot wear at all, and others that fit me like a glove. Obviously, I gravitate toward those designers. Getting specific about designers and their fit models may be overdoing it a bit, but you don't have to stress out about this. It really comes down to learning why something works or doesn't work for your shape. You should also consider how something *feels* as well as how it looks, so when you try on clothes, practice lots of different movements to make sure they move naturally with you. Don't be afraid to bust a move at the Gap!

I want to make a note here about larger sizes. When women (and sometimes men) feel large, they tend to try to hide their shape by wearing oversize black, draping clothes. I often made this mistake years ago when I was trying to hide my extra weight with big tops! This is worse than choosing form-fitting clothes, because baggy clothes give you a large, boxy, shelf- or tent-like shape. When clothes don't fit the shape of the body, the viewer's eyes fill in the rest, and they usually fill in more than is really there! Clothes with a more form-fitting shape are a better choice, believe it or not, and you certainly don't want to keep hiding in extra-large sizes as you start to lose weight.

The key is to keep observing and experimenting with lots of trial and error. Not only can this be fun, it's also very rewarding when it all comes together and you truly find your own personal style.

Wrapping It Up!

- Like it or not, people *do* judge you by your demeanor and style; developing your presentation is essential!

- Fear paralyzes your communication skills; experience develops them.

- Poorly developed communication skills prevent people from reaching their full potential in their careers and relationships.

- Good conversationalists are always in present time—in the moment.

- Ninety-three percent of what an audience gets from your message is based on you—your demeanor, delivery, and attitude.

- Only 7 percent of your message comes from the content of your speech.

- "Content without demeanor is like a hook without the bait."

- "It ain't what you say, it's the way that you say it."

- Audiences rarely retain more than three key points. Narrow yours down to two or three.

- Align yourself with the concern before you try to change a person's opinion.

- It's all about homework and preparation.

- Personal style is important because it tells people who you are, what you want, and what people should expect of you.

- Hair is the B Story!

- Aside from making you feel great and be healthier, a program of eating right and exercising regularly also gives you the benefit of looking good.

- Developing style comes from keen observation and lots of trial and error.

Nine

FALL IN LOVE WITH YOUR STRESS—OR IT WILL KILL YOU!

Wearing your life well is the same as wearing your reality well. A very common source of stress comes from trying to change what can't be changed, and especially from not *accepting* what can't be changed. For example, some people have a difficult time accepting their age. You should always strive to be your best and healthiest, and even though you're not going to stop the hands of time, you're not doomed to be the same forty-, fifty-, or seventy-year-old that your parents were at those ages. There's a lot of truth to statements like "Forty is the new thirty," but only if you are willing to make the transitions and move on gracefully to each stage of maturity by embracing it rather than fighting the reality of who you are. (Have you ever noticed that it's relatively common for sex symbols to die young?) The stress of aging, along with aging itself, takes its toll. I've noticed something interesting about comedians as well. Some have a difficult time accepting their reality, while other comedians embrace it. They seem to die either very young from self-destruction, as in the cases of Lenny Bruce, Freddie Prinze, John Belushi, Chris Farley, and Richard Jeni, or they live a long, full life, like George Burns and Bob Hope.

I've also found that if you miss a step along the way in your life, you're likely to just go back and live it anyway. You'll see this often in people who marry and have children young or have successful careers at a very young age. They tend to act out and behave like teenagers in their thirties, with alcohol abuse, smoking, sex, and drugs, because they didn't get to be wild back when they were young. Also, they are rarely emotionally or psychologically prepared for adulthood.

Choosing a Familiar . . . Misery

Change and the unfamiliar are very scary to most people. I remember one day in group therapy after everybody was whining about their problems, our therapist asked us to hypothetically put all our problems in the middle of the room and then take turns choosing the problem we would be most willing to solve. Without exception, each of us chose our original problem because it was the problem with which we were most familiar. It's easier to battle the familiar people, places, and other factors involved than it is to take on a completely new set of circumstances. People often feel that the unknown is much scarier even when the "known" is a disaster. At least it's a *familiar* disaster. We think to ourselves, "I know this stinks, but at least I know how to deal with this garbage!"

We all know people who move through life easily with a smile on their face no matter how challenging their life appears to be. They're always processing their problems in a positive way. If they hear about trouble on the horizon, they usually handle it like, "Oh, that's no big deal. I've already got six plates spinning. What difference will it make if I have seven?" They never seem to have a problem with one more kid, one more responsibility, or one more obligation to take care of. They don't expect everything to run smoothly, and when it doesn't, they aren't thrown by it.

Then there are those people whose lives could be going relatively well, but you'd never know it because they are always whining and complaining that they're overwhelmed and that their lives are more complicated and harder than anyone else's. And whenever you try to help someone like this, they discount your advice. If you say something like, "Oh, I know what that's like. Let me help you. When that happened to me, I . . ." they often interrupt by saying, "No, you can't help. This is different! You don't know what I'm going through!"

These people don't really *want* help. They don't really want a solution to their problem because they've actually grown to *like* having an enormous cross to bear. You want to say to them, "Well, who set it up to make it so difficult? For whom are you living this impossible life?" Even if you simplified their lives, they would still make it difficult. They really don't want solutions, because once there's a solution, they no longer have a problem to complain about.

A lot of this has to do with people's expectations. If you grow up with the expectation that life is easy, you will be shocked when you find out that it's not. If your mother greeted you every morning with homemade waffles and freshly squeezed orange juice while Bambi and Thumper dressed you in your robe and slippers, you are destined to be disappointed the rest of your life. Parents do much more damage when they overindulge their little princes and princesses. Life is tough! It begins as a struggle, going all the way back to the sperm and egg.

And we continue to compete for survival until the day we die. If you expect life to be easy, it becomes that much harder. But if you plan ahead, make frequent and necessary adjustments, and cope logically with obstacles, bumps, and detours, life can be wonderful and even easy.

It's essential, however, that you wake up with an attitude of "I love the smell of life in the morning!"

Far too many people greet their day as if it's a huge burden to contend with. Sometimes they even stress out in their dreams throughout the night. I have a good friend like this, who, ironically, also happens to be very successful (even though he feels like a failure most of the time). He's doing well despite his perpetually negative outlook; his success probably stems more from being driven by revenge. It may be working for him in one sense, but it's incredibly stressful in the long run. Not for a second is it a recipe for a happy, rewarding life. After years of dealing with his negativity, I finally told him that the message he sends to people every day is that no one understands him, he is the low man on the totem pole (even though he's not), and (as he always reminds me) if he didn't have bad luck he'd have no luck at all. I told him that everything he says feeds into this attitude and eventually he'll convince everyone around him that he's a broken-down man doomed to bad luck!

We all need to take stock in ourselves with this in mind. Even if everyone sees you as a brilliant talent, they won't want to hire you, recommend you, or choose you to be part of their team (or even date you!) if they consciously or unconsciously see you as a loser. When it comes to success, talent is actually less important than reliability and a winning attitude. I once was pitched an idea by a very charismatic, handsome young man. I was all ready to sign a deal with him until he told my manager, Rory Rosegarten, that he was really excited and optimistic about working with me because his last seven projects had failed. Rory instantly changed his opinion of the guy, and in good conscience, couldn't recommend my signing the deal.

Honesty is one thing, but sometimes it is much wiser to withhold information (or at least give it a positive spin), especially in (0–7) situations like that. Never say self-deprecating things to be funny, such as "I can't even get arrested in this town!" It's not worth the laugh. This kind of attitude eventually becomes a self-fulfilling prophecy. There's no reward for correctly predicting your own failure.

To be prepared for the struggle and stress of daily life, it's very important to be able to absorb, metabolize, and cope with negative setbacks. Everyone needs some sort of release valve to relieve the pressure that builds up from dealing with the stumbling blocks. For me it's exercise. Find the release valve that works for you—but make sure it's not destructive in itself. Alcohol can work as a release valve for a short time, but it becomes a much greater problem and stress than the initial problem it was meant to fix. Food, sex, and other drugs are also commonly used as release valves. These always intensify the original problem. You're not resolving the resistance or stress in life; you're creating something much bigger. You're swallowing a dog to catch the cat, because you swallowed a cat to catch the mouse, and the mouse to catch the spider, and whatever else they say in that kindergarten song!

Forget about the negative stress relievers and adopt the positive ones, starting with my favorite of all—exercise! Exercise is especially great because it can also be adopted as a hobby—defined as anything that you get lost in or take pride in simply for the pleasure of doing it. Hobbies are another category of positive stress reliever. Exercise hobbies such as ballroom dancing, tap, tennis, aerobics, golf, and swimming give twice the benefit as nonexercise hobbies such as gardening, collecting, and crafting. These are also great and recommended, but try to adopt a hobby that involves movement and exercise.

It's important to find the "juice" in everything you do throughout your day. Look for those little things, those little spark plugs that keep you going. Love and passion are great energizers and stress relievers. You can invest your heart into your spouse and kids, for example. One of my favorite parts of my day is driving my kids to school in the morning. To balance the stress of work, you can say, "I worked hard today, so I'm going to have a nice dinner with my kids tonight." Or, "Right after my busy season at work, I'm going to plan a nice weekend getaway with my family."

Another great stress reliever is meditation, and I'm not just talking about the usual Eastern meditation, in which you focus quietly. The meditation I prefer is organizing something in my house, whether it's a closet, drawer, or cabinet. It may seem a little oddball, but organizing something has always been wonderful therapy for me. It keeps me focused and gives me a steady rhythm, and I can actually feel the pressure releasing from my body. It's the same feeling I get when I walk on the treadmill.

We all have our own little idiosyncrasies and short fuses when it comes to stress and the things that bother us. My brother and coauthor, Lorin, for example, has a problem with noise. He becomes a crabby old man (even though he still looks thirty) when he hears a dog barking incessantly or a neighbor playing loud music. As you might guess, I have a problem with things disorganized and out of place. I can almost feel physically ill when my house or closet is a mess. But with two kids and a busy schedule, it's impossible to keep my house the way I like it to be. I have learned to put this "stress factor" aside. When I have to, I can ignore little messes around me by focusing on what is important rather than dwelling on something that I know in my heart to be trivial.

A very common stress factor for people these days is traffic. It no longer matters where you live; traffic is major drama everywhere. You can fight and stress out over a problem you can't really fix, or you can adopt ways to cope with it. If you don't, these little things in life can add up slowly over the years to kill you—or, in the case of road rage, kill you quickly! Remember, you can choose a different route, leave earlier, calm yourself down with breathing exercises, or listen to your favorite music, audio lectures, books on tape, or talk radio—whatever it takes to gain control of your anger over the traffic situation.

Here are a few other common stress makers and suggestions on how to embrace them or cope with them. Everything mentioned here is worth investigating so that you can try to remove the stress producers and live your life the way you want.

Messiness. People who've read my books know one of my all-time favorite tips about organization: Never leave a room empty-handed. If you follow it, you'll rarely be stressed about your home being messy again. I learned this great tip from my mother (who learned it from Ingrid Bergman in a fan magazine). I rarely saw her leave a room without picking something up, and I'm just like her now. In fact, I have my kids and husband doing this too. It's amazing how much work gets done automatically as a result. And you'll be much less stressed about mess!

Money. If money (or lack of it) is causing you stress, you need to examine first why you're having a financial problem. Have you been doing what you know you need to do to improve your situation? Debt dramas can only be resolved by facing the truth, assessing the damage, making a plan, and then sticking to it. It can be that simple. It does, however, require discipline. When I was a sophomore in college, my perception of money changed forever when a friend taught me how to respect money and stick to a budget. She made me write down everything I made and everything I spent, right down to the penny. Even though my income and expenditures have changed a lot since then, I still follow my friend's basic principles. Keep in mind that getting out of debt can be a fun and very satisfying project! Start out by assessing the damage, creating a plan of action, and then tracking your progress along the way.

Weight. Weight issues can be remedied in a similar way to fixing an unhealthy budget. Both require discipline, and both require a solid plan. As I've said elsewhere in this book and in others, weight reduction is all about improving the *quality* of your food—and the quantity will take care of itself. It never hurts to repeat that the key factor in getting healthy and controlling your weight is learning to love the food that loves you. Change your palate, and you change your life. I say this often because that's what it's all about!

Job. If you dread going into work every day, you need to figure out what's at the root of your anxiety. Once that's established, you can then try to remedy your stress. Is it the people you work with? Are you getting the respect you deserve? The right salary for your services? How is your work space set up? Is it disorganized? Get to the bottom of these questions, and you'll be on your way to resolving your stress—you can begin working toward a solution to reverse your problems.

Family Dramas. I'm always saying that the family structure works like a mobile. The weight and significance of each mobile piece is different. A family member's piece can be any combination of small, large, heavy, or light. Anytime a member goes through a change, whether it's illness, changing schools, leaving home, puberty, losing weight, losing a job, or greater success, the balance of these pieces tends to shift. That's why you'll see minor rebellions in the family dynamic whenever something new enters the picture. The trouble spots are not always obvious, but you can sense that something is causing unresolved stress. (Has it become such a regular part of your stress that you no longer remember the origin or cause?) At times, we're so used to a certain kind of stress that we no longer see it as stressful. If pain exists long enough, it stops feeling painful. Often we need to step away from our routine to see it as it really is, or someone new enters the picture and points it out to us.

Does some of your stress originate from the way your family relates to the rest of the world? Do you have any spooky family idiosyncrasies that have kept you from living more freely? Have you inherited some irrational family fears about flying, swimming, or dating? These unwanted fears can become stressful because people often want to live their lives in contrast from how they were raised, but some ignorant deep-rooted family fear is subconsciously stopping them. Lorin and I recently went to our elementary school reunion, and one of the local guys from our neighborhood said to Lorin, rather inappropriately, "I never went to your mom's dancing school because I always thought it was kind of gay."

And Lorin said to him, "I always got a kick out of guys like you. Because you were so worried about looking gay, you missed the opportunity to dance with, exercise with, and, most important, socialize with all the pretty girls in the neighborhood at our dancing school. Instead, you probably spent your time at the school gym working out with a bunch of sweaty guys!" This is a good example of the conflict between doing what you might want to do and being held back by some deep-rooted family fear. Don't be afraid to question something you have been following blindly all your life, especially when it feels wrong. It may be a source of stress because you never examined it from the other side. It's possible that the importance your family has been putting on an issue is no longer true or as important for you.

Relationships. If you've got stress in a romantic relationship, chances are that you're both feeding into it and causing stress for each other. Relationship stress is a two-way street. You can usually tell a lot about your relationship with someone by how you feel about yourself right after you've been with him or her. If you feel good, strong, and optimistic, that's an excellent indication that your relationship is healthy. If you feel belittled, resentful, or angry most of the time, you've got problems that need correcting. If they can't be corrected, the relationship should probably dissolve, unless your mutual combativeness is actually a source of stimulation for both of you, rather than a source of stress. Some people love to fight with each other; it's their foreplay. It may appear to outsiders to be stressful, but to the couple it isn't. What would kill one relationship actually fuels another. For example, my sister and her husband are world-class bridge players. They thrive on the competition of playing with and against each other in major tournaments around the world. Most other couples would probably want to kill each other over a game that is competitive with so much at stake, but not them. They met and happily married years ago, and their connection to the bridge world is one of the cornerstones of their relationship.

One quality I've observed in the world's greatest doubles partnerships in professional tennis is that each partner is constantly supporting the other. You could put the number-one- and number-two-ranked tennis players in the world on the same doubles team, and if they tend to be adversarial, they probably won't survive the first round at Wimbledon or the U.S. Open. But if you take two players ranked in the forties or fifties with great chemistry who are supporting each other's strengths and protecting each other's weaknesses, they'll have a great chance of winning the whole championship.

A big source of stress for many relationships is trust. Most people have a deep-rooted fear of being left in the dark when their partner is having an affair. It usually bothers people more when they find out they were cheated on after the fact than to know about the affair while it's going on! It gives them a little more sense of control over the situation—at least no one is pulling the wool over their eyes. People just hate feeling duped. This is a problem for women, but it seems that men in particular are bothered by deception. It can be a major blow to a man's ego and can be a significant source of stress.

Don't Be a Lemming

More than ever these days it is important to question authority and mistrust the information we're bombarded with day after day. A very discouraged friend of mine recently told me he'd read an article that claimed people ultimately can't change 80 percent of who they are, and that most attempts to change patterns of past failure are futile. I'm always amused by articles and claims like this, but I'm also angered, because people believe them. You can read all the stats you want, but what matters most is your belief system in *yourself*!

Keep in mind the purpose behind what you see, read, and hear in the media. Information is dispersed in order to sell magazines, or advertising space, or some other product that's often unknown to the reader. The media need to grab your attention, even if in order to do so they say things that defy logic and common sense. Sometimes the results that come out of very extensive research projects turn out to be bogus, because they're funded and driven by an industry that profits from predetermined results. It's very common for competing industries to reach completely different conclusions, even though both did extensive research. Both can't be right. In fact, often both are wrong! If the public is confused about the conflicting information they get, it's because the information is *meant* to confuse you. We have become a research-obsessed society, which is ironic because so much of it is bogus. Contradicting results are common, so we know at least *one* of them has to be false! Yet people will spout about some study as if it were the final word on an issue.

Be especially skeptical when you hear favorable information about the pharmaceutical or meat and dairy industries. The meat and dairy industries were major players behind the creation of the confusing government food pyramids, both in the early nineties and more recently. These pyramids are intentionally confusing and misleading, because if the public truly understood the dangers of eating animal protein on a daily basis, there would be a substantial reduction in its consumption, and those industries would be harmed. Whenever a report comes out citing the dangers of animal products, another report, secretly connected to the meat and dairy industry, shows some kind of benefit associated with eating meat and dairy.

As I mentioned earlier, I was campaigning for a greater awareness of the dangers of meat and dairy products in Washington at the time the latest food pyramid was being created. I learned how futile it can be when you're up against a rich and powerful group like the meat and dairy industry. The pharmaceutical companies, who are also in the business of misinformation, want the world to believe that optimal health depends on pills manufactured in a lab. They propagate information that almost completely downplays the role diet and exercise play in preventing and curing disease. Unfortunately, because the pharmaceutical companies fund much of the education and textbooks of our medical schools, the information disseminated to our doctors is based on the same philosophy and misinformation. It is not uncommon for a patient to be discharged from a hospital with nine or ten prescriptions, instead of what would really help his or her long-term health and prospects: a recommendation for a strict regimen of a nutrient-dense diet and exercise to stimulate and fortify the immune system along with the other systems (cardiovascular, endocrine, and circulatory).

Skepticism is your greatest tool in the battle against misinformation. When I read books on pregnancy before my first child, I saw all the common warnings: You'll gain X amount of weight, you'll suffer from frequent bouts of edema, bloating, and constipation, and so on. When I researched it myself, I realized that the dairy-enriched diet that was commonly recommended with this advice was what *caused* all of these negative symptoms.

You cannot be a lemming and just blindly follow everyone, statistics, or the opinion of the majority. Sometimes you have to trust your instincts, even when they go against what 90 percent of the population is telling you. There's a small percentage of the population that stands to make great profits by misleading the majority. Never be afraid to go against the tide. Revolutionary thinking is almost always behind true progress in life.

Wrapping It Up!

- A very common source of stress comes from trying to change what can't be changed, or not *accepting* what can't be changed.

- Change and the unfamiliar are very scary to most people.

- Far too many people greet their day as a burden.

- To be prepared for the struggle and stress of daily life, it's very important to be able to absorb, metabolize, and cope with negative setbacks.

- You can stress out over a problem you can't really fix, or you can adopt ways to cope with it.

- Deep debt can be resolved only by facing the truth.

- When you focus on the *quality* of your food, the *quantity* takes care of itself.

- If you dread going into work every day, you need to figure out what's at the root of your anxiety.

- Family structures work like a mobile. Every piece affects the whole arrangement.

- We can get so used to some kinds of stress that we no longer see them as stressful.

- You can usually tell a lot about your relationship with someone by how you feel about yourself right after you've been with him or her.

- Most people have a deep-rooted fear of being left in the dark when their partner is having an affair.

- It is more important than ever to question authority and mistrust information.

- It's very common for competing industries to reach completely different conclusions in their research. Both can't be right.

- Never be a lemming!

Ten

THE SEXIEST ORGAN IS . . .
YOUR BRAIN!

You knew I would save the best for (almost) last!

It seems that no matter what other topic women (or men) start to discuss, sooner or later the subject always gets around to our favorite one . . . sex! It's such an interesting subject, and talking about it is like singing karaoke. People are reluctant to start, but once they do, there's no stopping them.

In doing research on the subject of passion, energy, and lust, I've come to realize that, more than anything else, your sexiest organ is your brain! That's it. That's the center.

Your brain makes or breaks everything you do in your life. Perception is everything! No matter how negative something feels right now, your perception can be altered so that you can better understand, accept, enjoy, eat, behave, and ultimately feel so much better than you do. Your brain determines how you respond to pain, fear, comfort, and pleasure. Anyone who has done my Total Health Makeover program knows how different you can feel about food after eating healthy for a while. There are many things I used to love to eat that I would never touch now, and many foods that I wouldn't have found tasty in the past that I now love. There is a vast difference between my old palate and my new healthy palate. This "doing a 180" is possible not just for food, but for most things in life, especially *sex*!

Every feeling about sex starts in that potent brain of yours. It's connected to how you feel about yourself, what you've observed in your parents and their relationship, and what they've taught you about the opposite sex. It's about how you relate to your siblings, peers, and former lovers, and even about what you've learned from religion, the media, politics, and the other messages you're exposed to every day. All this information can muddle your clarity and self-confidence when it comes to sex. You can't just run around reacting instinctively like other animals (no matter how much fun that seems), but at least you have the ability to spice things up with your own creativity. Dogs and cats aren't doing a lot of dress-up and foreplay. (Except for Snoopy, who always struck me as a bit of a . . . well . . . *dog*!)

You can't wear your life well if you don't feel comfortable with your own sexuality. It's as simple as that. It doesn't matter what other people say about you; how *you* feel in own your skin controls your sex life. We've all known some incredibly sexy people who deep down feel very *unsexy*. You could look like Angelina Jolie, but if you've got problems in your head, you've got problems in the bedroom. (Then again, if you look like Angelina Jolie, your partner probably doesn't care if you're a nut job.)

Nothing makes us feel more alive than a fun, exhilarating, naughty and bawdy sex life! We're all capable of surrendering ourselves to great passion and wild abandon, and there's nothing wrong with that. We should allow ourselves the freedom to drop our guard and explore. But there's no doubt about it: The biggest mood killer is self-consciousness. You can't be a good lover if your "attention units" are focused on the negative. Whether it's body issues for women (weight, small breasts, chubby thighs) or body issues for men (penis size, beer belly, excessive sweating), on stage or in the bedroom, anxiety can keep even the most confident and gifted players worrying about their "performance."

Sex is not the most important part of an intimate relationship, but if it's "off," it can *become* the most important part. I know many women who say they "live in their heads" when it comes to sex. Their imaginations are sexually charged and fertile with creativity and longings, but their partners have no idea because these women are silent.

Too afraid to open their mouths.
Too afraid of their own rage.
Too afraid of their own power.

They keep their hunger and fantasies to themselves. This eventually leads to trouble because their partners sense an estrangement and feel left out. Don't ever expect your partner to be a mind reader. There's nothing to be gained by keeping your longings and passions to yourself. Women are often afraid to express their real desires because they fear their lover will judge them as being too loose or too kinky. You might be surprised to find that your partner really appreciates your wild side. My advice is to introduce these feelings and fantasies a little at a time and pay attention to how your partner responds. There's no point in rushing this. In fact, it's fun to pace yourself, let it evolve slowly, and build some sexual tension.

Much of what we think about sex, lust, and passion generates from early impressions of our parents and how they related to each other. These early imprintings still hold power over us, whether we like it or not. Images of seeing them together, relating to each other, their body language, and physical comfort or discomfort with each other all factor in. We also have images from movies, of course, and what we think a relationship should be like in terms of behavior and physical appearance for each person. From the moment we first stepped into the dating arena, we've had expectations, influenced by how people respond to us and how awkward or confident we felt compared to our parents' relationship and those we saw on film. (Believe me, to this day, I'm still trying to live up to every image from the 1967 version of *The Thomas Crown Affair*!) So here you are, with all this "baggage" from your past. All the dating, good and bad. All the relationships, good and bad. All the heartbreak you've been through and have seen in other people. All the *sex* you've had, good and bad. All the *body issues*!

This is what you're bringing to bed with you—in your head. It's way too crowded in there! It's like a Coen brothers film. It's like Cinemax after midnight. And it's not just limited to the bedroom—you bring these images to every relationship and encounter you have. It's amazing that your head doesn't explode!

And then, to really complicate things . . . the *other* person has all *their* baggage! No wonder it's hard to get frisky.

On top of all that, you also have your day, your kids, your life, your job, and all the other "stuff"—the anger, resentment, indifference, and button-pushing—that you might be feeling toward the other person. Add on boredom and hostility, and it's not surprising that most of us want to have a drink or some other mood-altering substance in order to turn off our brains and anesthetize ourselves to get into another state of mind. This often leads to a dangerous downward spiral and fighting or avoiding thoughts that can make them even stronger. Instead of trying to shut out or mask what's bothering you, focus on the good stuff, the fun, exciting pleasures. If the other more negative stuff creeps in, so what? Don't dwell on it or let it bother you. Accept it and get back to what you enjoy.

Thinking Sexy

"Thinking sexy" is a state of mind you should carry throughout your day, not just when it's time to go to bed. Whatever the dramas from your past, your body issues, your everyday life issues, and all your other negative sexual issues, you can still *think* sexy. It's okay to have all your feelings, but try not to let them take you to the dark side. People often focus on their negative sexual past, and this leads to unhealthy sexual energy. Dwelling on the negative does no one any good—not you and not your partner. Realize that you are human, and the people you may resent from your past are also just human and susceptible to all the usual human weaknesses. Forgive yourself and them and move on.

Never focus on your liabilities, *especially* in the bedroom. Face the fact that everybody has them. Guys are usually much less self-conscious, so they're unaware of all the little things that make us crazy about ourselves. Women see themselves naked and notice all their imperfections. Men see us naked and think, "Yippee, she's naked!" Most men don't sweat the details. I always say that if men felt about women the way women feel about themselves, we would probably die out as a species.

If people could get their "attention units" off themselves and onto their partners, they'd have a much better time and feel much sexier. In other words, stop wasting time thinking about what you don't bring to the party; focus instead on what you do best. It could be something physical, like an especially sexy body part of yours, or some kind of exciting technique, or even a creative fantasy you'd love to share. The same goes for how you feel about your partner. Don't focus on what you don't like about him. We all have something we excel in. Remind yourself about the things that attracted you to him in the first place. Most important, keep your receptors open to discovering new things that may be attractive about him *now*. When you make your partner feel desirable, he or she will sense this and automatically *become* more desirable. A relationship can feed on itself in a positive, complementary, mutually ego-supporting direction, or it can spiral downward in a negative, self-conscious, defensive, competitive path. It's up to you. You have the power to lead it in the direction you want.

The Pleasure Principle

Have you ever been lucky enough to have a partner who thoroughly enjoyed the whole "ritual" of sex, the kind of person who treats sex like a ten-course gourmet feast, with lots of pleasure peaks and valleys along the way? When I've been involved in a relationship like that (like now with my husband!), I always get excited just thinking about what our next encounter will be like. I find myself developing creative little ideas to bring to the "dining" experience!

I've found that you don't have to wait around hoping to get together with that kind of person. You don't have to wait for anyone to give you permission to be sexy! You can take the lead and become that person yourself, and most partners will be thrilled to follow you. Some may require a little more time and clever coaxing, but be patient. It's always worth it. Never feel inhibited about role-playing, dressing up, playing games, or exploring secret fantasies. This is about pleasure! As long as both partners are into it, you should allow yourself the freedom to go wherever your fantasies take you. That's when you can truly surprise yourself.

A big part of being healthy and wearing your life well is being in touch with your body. Feeling alive and vibrant and comfortable in your own skin is something worth shooting for! A popular exercise I assign in my classes is to spend the whole day or a weekend thinking sexy. This is nothing to be afraid of—it just helps you get in touch with the fact that your sexuality stems from that sexy brain of yours. Don't be afraid to take it a step beyond thinking and try wearing something sexy or acting sexy. It can be about donning lingerie, doing something for your significant other, or learning something new about yourself. Believe me, thinking of yourself as a sensuous person makes you feel alive, gives you energy, gets the juices flowing, and makes every cell in your body stand at attention.

A sexual relationship is what separates you and your partner from the rest of the world. No one else knows what goes on behind closed doors, but it really is the laboratory for your relationship. It's the one thing the two of you don't share with anyone else in the world. And it shouldn't be! It's not just about the sex act, either. It's about being close. It's about sharing and intimacy. It's about "toasty time" and downloading the rest of your day. It's about so much. And that's why it's so loaded.

Whenever I hear people tell me that they're bored in bed, I say what my mother always said: "If you're bored, you're boring!" This is especially true when it comes to sex. People often blame their partner when they really should be analyzing what *they're* not bringing to the bedroom. You may be thinking, "This all sounds great, but I've been with my partner for so many years, and he does this and I do that, and he's not very good." You have the power to change that, but you've got to shake up the routine a little. Instead of thinking about what he's *not* doing, focus more on how sexy *you* can be. Start to see yourself as this sexual creature that *you* are bringing to the otherwise boring bedroom! He doesn't even have to know that you're getting off on this idea. Give yourself permission to think whatever you want. And for those of you who complain that sex is the only thing your partner wants to share: Maybe it's the only way he knows how to express himself. You can work up to what you want and need from him, but try changing yourself and your perceptions first. (Wasn't it John F. Kennedy who said, "Ask not what your partner can do for you—ask what you can do for your partner"?)

The next time you get together with your partner (it doesn't matter if it's a long-term relationship or someone you just starting dating) as a little experiment, spend the day "thinking" sexy. Move differently in your body as you walk through your office. Wear something that feels good or shows off your best body part. Make a phone call and say something a little more provocative than you usually do. Take five minutes out of your day and daydream about the best sexual experience you ever had. Even better, plan a sexy scenario for you and your partner with as much consideration and forethought as you would an important dinner party. What if just you, and you alone, had this delicious little secret? Forget about all your imperfections, your issues with your life and partner, and just spend some serious creative time indulging your fantasies. There are many ways we can change ourselves so that by the time we hit those sheets (or the kitchen table!) there's a lot more going on than the same old, same old!

Most people assume that being sexy requires another person. That's always nice, of course, but try to inspire a feeling of sexiness from your own self-worth and self-expression. Carrying yourself with confidence is sexy. Feeling feminine and sensuous in your clothing is sexy. Being assertive and powerful is sexy for men *and* women. Walking with purpose is sexy. Breaking a sweat is sexy. Being clean is sexy. Sleeping peacefully is sexy.

Sex is so much about so many other things besides the sexual act. It's about being open-minded and seeing the possibilities in everything. It's about being sensual and sensuous. It's about eating a meal and really tasting it, really experiencing the flavors and the textures in your mouth and on your tongue, and really being able to smell and touch and take in everything that's around you. It's about being alive!

You know what's sexy? Anyone who is comfortable enough in his or her own body to just let go!

Wrapping It Up!

- Your sexiest organ is—your brain!

- Perception can be altered so that you can understand, accept, enjoy, eat, behave, and ultimately feel better than you do right now.

- You need to feel comfortable with your own sexuality.

- Nothing makes us feel more alive than a fun, exhilarating, serendipitously naughty, and bawdy sex life!

- Sex is not the most important part of an intimate relationship, but if it's "off," it can *become* the most important part.

- Don't ever expect your partner to be a mind reader.

- Much of what we think about sex, lust, and passion generates from early impressions of our parents and how they related to each other.

- "Thinking sexy" is a state of mind to carry throughout your day, not just at bedtime.

- Convert your negative "attention units" of yourself into positive attention on your partner.

- Stop wasting time thinking about your liabilities; focus instead on what you do best.

- When you make your partner feel desirable, your partner will automatically *become* more desirable.

- A relationship can feed on itself in a positive, complementary, mutually ego-supporting direction, or it can spiral downward in a negative, self-conscious, defensive, competitive path.

- You don't have to wait for anyone's permission to be sexy!

- A big part of being healthy and wearing your life well is being in touch with your body.

- A sexual relationship is what separates you and your partner from the rest of the world.

- "If you're bored, you're boring!" This is especially true when it comes to sex.

- Instead of thinking about what your partner's *not* doing, focus more on how sexy *you* can be.

- Ask not what your partner can do for you—ask what you can do for your partner.

- Plan a sexy scenario for you and your partner.

- Don't be afraid to "think sexy" throughout your day.

Eleven

THE BOOTY CAMP BLITZ

By now you probably have a pretty good idea of how to wear your life well, but even with all this knowledge, you might sometimes need that little five-day push to get you to a fast-approaching deadline—think wedding, high school reunion, or job interview. This is the Booty Camp Blitz, and it's just the trick to getting a better body in five short days. The Booty Camp Blitz is the little ace in your back pocket that you can play at any time. Try it once, and you'll know it works!

> *What fun! Five days of mini-meals, extra workouts, and daily challenges can really jump-start (or restart!) healthy habits and make a difference in your health, even in that short time. A bit of competition along the way adds to the fun and camaraderie of the class.*
>
> —LYRICAL,
> Marilu.com
> member

BOOTY CAMP BLITZ 5-DAY CONTRACT

The Booty Camp Rules

1. **Show up to play!** Throw yourself into this for the entire 5 days.

2. **Skin brush**—every day, before your exercise or shower (see pages 78–79 for instructions).

3. **Drink water**—a minimum of half your body weight in ounces each day (or 100 ounces max if heavier than 200 pounds).

4. **Eat single serving portions**—small meals—so that you don't stretch your stomach. Follow the list of Booty Camp menu choices that starts on page 207.

5. **NO dairy products, no red meat, no refined sugar, and no alcohol** for all 5 days.

6. **Eat organic** whenever possible.

7. **All salads served with** a nondairy dressing (recipes follow), lemon squeeze, or no dressing at all.

8. **Grill fish, chicken breast, or tofu** with either no oil or a light spray of oil.

9. **For weight-loss purposes**, your mini-meals should not include more than 2 servings of whole-grain pasta, brown rice, or potato in any given day. It's best if you eat no more than 5 meals with carbs during the Booty Camp Blitz.

10. **Stop eating 3 hours or more before bedtime.**

11. **All teas are decaffeinated, no sweeteners added.** Choose chamomile for tranquility, peppermint for digestion, red clover for energy, and burdock root for weight loss.

12. **All juices are 100 percent, no sweeteners added.** Choose carrot, celery, spinach, beet, or any combination of these. If you choose to drink fruit juices (apple, orange, grapefruit, pomegranate, and so on), be sure to dilute by half with water.

13. **Take baking soda baths every evening** that you can manage to fit them in!

14. **Exercise at least 30 minutes every day** of this program. Don't be afraid to challenge yourself!

15. **Gimme 5 mini-workouts**—choose 5 of these workouts to complete every day in addition to your required 30 minutes of exercise.

- Jog or run—5 minutes
- Weights—5 sets of 5 arm curls, shoulder lifts, or knee lifts
- Play an active game with a kid (such as H-O-R-S-E tag, or Frisbee)
- Swim—5 laps in pool
- Resistance bands—5 sets of 5 arm curls, chest flies, or shoulder lifts
- Jump rope or hula hoop—5 minutes
- Crunches—5 sets of 20
- Push-ups—5 sets of 5
- Pilates/yoga—5 minutes just before bed
- Dancing—5 minutes around the house
- Stairs—5 flights a day
- Walk—5 blocks

16. Get a good night's sleep every night!

I, _____, do hereby agree to fol-
low the Booty Camp Rules and Eating Plan for 5 consecutive days
and keep a daily log of my progress.

Dated _____

BOOTY CAMP BLITZ—GIMME 5!
5-DAY MENU

- Select 5 mini-meals from the menu each day. An asterisk denotes that the recipe is included here.

- Space your meals no more than 3 hours apart—for example, 6 am–9 am–12 noon–3 pm–6 pm.

- Leave 12 hours between the last meal of the day and your breakfast the following day.

- 1 serving of fruit=1 medium apple, orange, or pear; ½ banana; ½ cup cut fruit (about the size of a tennis ball).

- 1 serving of vegetable=1 cup leafy; ½ cup cooked or raw.

- 3 ounces of protein=the size of a deck of cards.

- 1 serving of cooked pasta or grains=approximately the size of your fist.

- Salads may be served with 2 teaspoons of Dressing 101*, Dressing 102*, or other healthy low-fat nondairy dressing.

- Eat whole-grain bread dry or with avocado or soy margarine.

- Limit yourself to no more than *one* mini-meal latte, cookie, or ice-cream "treat" per day.

- Limit yourself to no more than *two* restaurant meals during the five days. Be sure to follow the Booty Camp Rules (no dairy products, no red meat, no refined sugar, and no alcohol).

- Eat slowly. Allow your brain to receive the signal that you're full, which usually takes about 20 minutes.

Booty Camp Menu

Select five of the following menu choices each day. See the appendix on page 249 for more information on food combining—but I've planned these mini-meals so that each is properly food combined, so no worries!

1. **Fruit** (2 servings)

2. **Fruit** 1 serving acid fruit (grapefruit, orange, strawberries, cranberries, kiwi, or pineapple) eaten with 10 plain almonds

3. **Fruit salad** 2 cups of diced fresh fruits (except sweet fruits such as bananas, plantains, dates, persimmons, figs, prunes, raisins, or dried fruit)

4. **Oatmeal** (½ cup dry), cooked with ½ teaspoon honey, stevia, agave, or maple syrup

5. **Whole-wheat toast** (1 slice) or whole-grain waffle (1) topped with sugar-free peanut butter (1 tablespoon) and honey (½ tablespoon)

6. **Scrambled egg whites** (2), with 1 slice whole-grain flourless toast

7. **Simple Spinach Soup*** (12 ounces) with 2 cups mixed greens salad or 1 slice whole-grain flourless toast

8. **Joey's "Chicken" Soup*** with 2 cups mixed greens salad or 1 slice whole-grain flourless toast

9. **Creamy Daikon Soup*** with 2 cups mixed greens salad or 1 slice whole-grain flourless toast

10. **Mixed greens salad** (2 cups) with ½ cup warm brown rice, 1 diced Roma tomato, and 6 olives

11. **Mixed greens salad** with ½ cup legumes such as soybeans, black beans, pinto beans, garbanzo beans, or lentils

12. **Warm Veggie Salad***

13. **Grilled Vegetable Salad*** with 3 ounces protein, such as salmon, snapper, chicken breast, or grilled tofu

14. **Japanese Baby Greens Salad*** (2 cups) with a whole-grain roll

15. **Salad with Beets***

16. **Balsamic Marinated Beets*** served over 2 cups salad greens

17. **Salade Niçoise***

18. **Taco Salad***

19. **Tuna and Asparagus Salad***

20. **Tuna-lettuce wraps or chicken-lettuce wraps** lettuce wrapped around ½ cup tuna salad or chicken salad made with Vegenaise

21. **Tuna salad or chicken salad** (½ cup tuna mixed with 1 teaspoon Nayonaise or Vegenaise) on a bed of lettuce with tomato and/or cucumber

22. **Nori Salad Wrap***

23. **Avocado:** (2 tablespoons) with tomato and cucumber slices on 1 slice whole-grain flourless bread

24. **Tomato and Basil Sandwich***

25. **ALT—Avocado, Lettuce, and Tomato Sandwich***

26. **Power Rice & Rye*** or brown rice (½ cup) with 12 ounces of soup (using menu item 7, 8, or 9)

27. **Power Rice & Rye*** or brown rice (½ cup) with 2 cups mixed greens salad

28. **Steamed Veggies over Quinoa*** (½ cup cooked quinoa)

29. **Three-Grain Pilaf*** (½ cup) with 1 cup steamed spinach

30. **Angel Hair Pasta with Lemon and Garlic*** with 2 cups mixed greens salad

31. **Pasta Primavera*** with 2 cups mixed greens salad or 1 cup steamed fresh asparagus

32. **Pasta** (½ cup whole-wheat, spinach, corn, or rice pasta) with marinara sauce (no sugar added) and 1 cup veggies

33. **Pasta with Fresh Vegetable Tomato Sauce*** (½ cup pasta)

34. **Steamed veggies of your choice** (2 cups)

35. **Grilled Veggie Packets*** with 2 cups salad greens

36. **Corn on the cob** (1 ear) with 2 cups salad greens and 2 slices fresh tomato

37. **Baked Potato, Yam, or Sweet Potato with Marinated Vegetables***

38. **Green Beans with Pine Nuts*** with ½ cup brown rice or Power Rice & Rye*

39. **Sautéed Broccoli Rabe*** with ½ cup brown rice or Power Rice & Rye* (serve in nori wrap, if desired)

40. **Veggie pizza** ½ whole-wheat pita topped with nondairy cheese, tomatoes, avocados, and basil

41. **Vegetable and legume stir-fry** cooked with a maximum of 1 tablespoon oil and 2 cups veggies

42. **Eggless Salad*** on 1 slice whole-grain flourless bread

43. **Turkey patty** (4 ounces), grilled, with lettuce, tomato, and onion and served with 1 cup steamed spinach or broccoli

44. **Grilled or broiled chicken, fish, portobello mushroom, or tofu** (4 ounces) with 1 cup grilled, steamed, or raw vegetables or 2 cups mixed greens salad

45. **Roasted Chicken with Garlic and Rosemary*** with 2 cups mixed greens salad or 1 cup steamed fresh seasonal veggies

46. **Chinese-Style Steamed Fish*** (4 ounces) with 2 cups mixed greens salad

47. **Grilled Teriyaki Tofu or Fish*** (4 ounces) with 2 cups mixed greens salad

48. **Spicy Grilled Salmon (or Chicken)*** (4 ounces) with 2 cups mixed greens salad or 1 cup steamed fresh seasonal veggies

49. **Herb-Infused Whole Baked Fish*** (4 ounces) with 2 cups mixed greens salad or 1 cup steamed fresh seasonal veggies

50. **Classic Bruschetta*** (3 slices)

51. **Whole-wheat crackers** (12) spread with 2 teaspoons sugar-free peanut butter

52. **Salsa** (3/4 cup all-natural) with a handful of baked tortilla chips

53. **Air-popped popcorn** (2 cups) with spray of Bragg Liquid Aminos if desired

54. **Hummus** (1/2 cup) with a handful of baked tortilla chips

55. **Sweet Pea Guacamole*** (1/2 cup) with a handful of baked tortilla chips or 2 cups raw veggies

56. **Edamame** (3/4 cup)

57. **Vegan cookie** Uncle Eddie's (1), Alternative Baking Co. (½), or other healthy cookie without refined sugar

58. **Soy Delicious ice cream** (3/4 cup), vanilla, chocolate, or strawberry

59. **Fresh Fruit Sorbet*** (1 cup)

60. **Soy yogurt** (1 cup plain) topped with 1 teaspoon honey, 2 tablespoons granola, and ½ banana

61. **Iced soy decaf latte** (12 ounces)

BOOTY CAMP RECIPES

Simple Spinach Soup

MENU ITEM #7
SERVES 4

4 cups vegetable broth
½ cup chopped chard or kale
1 large carrot, sliced thin
1 ½ cups sliced mushrooms
2 cups fresh baby spinach

In a large pot over medium heat, bring the broth and chard to a boil for 3 to 5 minutes. Add the carrot and mushrooms. When the carrot is tender, add the spinach. Stir for about 5 seconds and it's done.

Joey's "Chicken" Soup—
Marilu's Vegan Version!

MENU ITEM #8

SERVES 4

4   quarts vegetable broth

½   large yellow onion, peeled and chopped

3   celery stalks, sliced

4   carrots, sliced (optional)

2   cups sliced mushrooms

2   cups cut green beans (fresh or frozen)

2   cups broccoli stems and tree tops

In a large pot over medium heat, bring the vegetable broth, onion, celery, and carrots (if using) to a boil. Turn the heat to medium-low and simmer about 5 minutes, or until the vegetables begin to soften. Add the mushrooms, green beans, and broccoli stems and cook 2 to 3 minutes. Turn off heat and stir in the broccoli tops.

Creamy Daikon Soup

from Healthy Life Kitchen

MENU ITEM #9

SERVES 6 TO 8

3 tablespoons soy margarine

2 cups finely chopped yellow onion

½ cup minced shallots

4 cups vegetable stock

2 long, large daikon radishes, peeled and cut into small pieces

Salt and pepper to taste

Melt the soy margarine in a heavy pot over low heat. Add the onion and shallots and cook, covered, until tender, about 5 minutes. Add the vegetable stock and daikon and bring to a boil over medium heat. Reduce the heat and simmer until the daikon is tender, about 20 minutes. Pour the soup through a strainer. Reserve the liquid and transfer the solids to a blender or food processor. Puree, adding small amounts of the reserved broth to help blend (not too much, or it could splash out and burn you). Place the puree back into the pot and stir in the reserved broth bit by bit until you've reached the desired consistency for your soup. Season to taste with salt and pepper.

Dressing 101

from The 30-Day Total
Health Makeover

SERVES 1

1 teaspoon olive oil
1 teaspoon balsamic, or white wine, or red wine vinegar
1 teaspoon Dijon mustard

In a small bowl, combine all ingredients and whisk well. Drizzle on top of your salad and toss.

Dressing 102

from The 30-Day Total
Health Makeover

SERVES 2

1 **tablespoon olive oil**
1 **teaspoon balsamic vinegar**
⅛ **teaspoon soy sauce**

In a small bowl, combine all ingredients and whisk well. Drizzle on
top of your salad and toss.

Warm Veggie Salad

MENU ITEM #12
SERVES 1

Salad

1 handful fresh green beans

1 carrot, sliced

1 teaspoon olive oil

1 small zucchini, halved lengthwise and sliced

½ small yellow onion, diced

2 cups salad greens

Dressing

2 teaspoons balsamic, red wine, or white wine vinegar

1 teaspoon olive oil

2 teaspoons Dijon mustard

1 teaspoon fresh parsley, chopped

Steam the green beans and carrot slices for 3 to 4 minutes. Heat a sauté pan over medium heat and add the olive oil. Add the green beans, carrot, zucchini, and onion and sauté for 3 minutes, until heated through and softened. In a small bowl, whisk together the dressing ingredients. Add the dressing to the vegetables, toss to coat, and remove from the heat. Serve on salad greens.

Grilled Vegetable Salad

MENU ITEM #13

SERVES 4

Salad

1 large red onion, peeled

1 zucchini

1 yellow squash

1 medium to large portobello mushroom

1 bunch (2 cups) arugula, rinsed

1 bunch (2 cups) mixed Asian greens, rinsed

Vinaigrette

4 tablespoons balsamic vinegar

2 teaspoons miso paste

1 teaspoon brown mustard

1 tablespoon water

1 tablespoon olive oil

In a medium bowl, whisk together all the vinaigrette ingredients. Brush the vinaigrette on the onion, zucchini, squash, and mushroom. Grill the veggies on all sides to your taste, 5 to 7 minutes or longer. Chop the veggies and serve immediately on top of the greens.

Japanese Baby Greens Salad

from Healthy Life Kitchen

MENU ITEM #14

SERVES 1

- 2 cups mixed baby greens, rinsed and dried carefully
- 1 teaspoon Sucanat
- ¾ tablespoon white wine vinegar
- ½ teaspoon sea salt
- ¼ teaspoon freshly ground pepper
- 2 tablespoons extra-virgin olive oil

Wash and dry the greens very well. In a bowl, whisk together Sucanat, vinegar, salt, and pepper. Drizzle in the oil, whisking until blended. Toss the dressing and lettuce together to lightly coat the greens.

Salad with Beets

MENU ITEM #15

SERVES 1

2 large or 3 medium beets with greens
1 serving Dressing 101 (see page 216)
2 cups salad greens

Scrub the beets and cut off most of the greens, leaving 1 inch of the greens and the root intact. Place in a pan of cold water to cover and bring to a simmer over medium-low heat. Simmer at least 50 minutes for 2-inch beets (longer for larger ones). Prick with a fork to see if they're done—but don't do it too early, because the color bleeds into the cooking water and we're trying to prevent that for as long as possible. When they're fork-tender, drain the beets and run cold water on them to cool them down. As soon as you can, slice off the top and the root of each beet and slip off the peel. Cut the beets into chunks and toss them with Dressing 101. Marinate for 20 to 30 minutes. Serve warm or cold over salad greens.

Balsamic Marinated Beets

MENU ITEM #16

SERVES 6

3   medium beets (¾ pound)
2   tablespoons balsamic vinegar
    Pinch of sea salt

Place the beets in a medium saucepan and cover with 1 inch of water. Cover the pot and simmer for about 1 hour, or until the beets are tender. Drain the beets and rinse under cool water to slip off the skins. Cut the beets in half, then cut each half into 3 wedges. Place in a bowl, toss with the balsamic vinegar, and sprinkle with salt. Serve immediately, or marinate for 30 minutes for more intense flavor.

Salade Niçoise

from The 30-Day Total
Health Makeover

MENU ITEM #17
SERVES 1

6   ounces grilled ahi tuna, or one 6-ounce can of tuna packed
    in water
2   cups mixed greens
1   tomato, chopped
    Handful of green beans, raw or steamed
2   hard-boiled egg whites (optional)

Dressing
1   tablespoon olive oil
1   teaspoon balsamic, white wine, or red wine vinegar
1   teaspoon Dijon mustard

In a small bowl, whisk together the dressing ingredients. Compose
the other ingredients on a plate and drizzle the dressing on top.

Taco Salad

MENU ITEM #18
SERVES 1

½ cup of your favorite beans, drained and rinsed

6 black olives, diced

1 Roma tomato, chopped

½ cucumber, chopped

2 cups lettuce of your choice

¼ cup salsa

Dash of hot sauce (optional)

Add the beans, olives, tomato, and cucumber to a bed of lettuce greens. Top with salsa. Sprinkle with a dash of hot sauce, if desired. Olé!

Tuna and Asparagus Salad

MENU ITEM #19
SERVES 1

Salad

4 to 6 ounces tuna, either Ahi or canned chunk light tuna (sear if using Ahi, crumble if canned tuna)

6 to 8 stalks asparagus, steamed or blanched in salted water, cut into bite-size pieces

2 cups mixed greens

Dressing

1 tablespoon Nayonaise

1 tablespoon Dijon mustard

½ teaspoon juice from a bottle of capers

1 tablespoon balsamic vinegar

Toss all the salad ingredients in a mixing bowl. In a small bowl, whisk together the dressing ingredients. Drizzle the dressing on top of the salad.

Nori Salad Wrap

MENU ITEM #22

SERVES 1

1 **sheet nori**
Leftover salad
Brown rice, if desired

Roll the nori into a triangle (or "sno-cone") and fill it with leftover salad. Add a little brown rice if you like. Two skinny wraps or one chunky wrap equals one serving.

Tomato and Basil Sandwich

MENU ITEM #24

SERVES 1

1 slice flourless bread

Roasted garlic (optional)

1 or 2 vine-ripened beefsteak tomatoes, sliced thick

1 or 2 basil leaves, torn

1 or 2 thin slices red onion

Splash of balsamic vinegar, or Dressing 101 or Dressing 102
(see pages 216 and 217).

If you have roasted garlic on hand, it's a superb addition to this recipe!
Just smash some of those cloves into the bread. Assemble the sandwich
as desired and top with a little balsamic vinegar or dressing.

Note: To brown-bag this, place the sliced tomatoes, onion, basil, and
dressing in a separate container. Assemble when ready to eat.

ALT—Avocado, Lettuce, and Tomato Sandwich

MENU ITEM #25

SERVES 1

1 slice flourless bread, toasted

2 tablespoons avocado

1 thick slice homegrown or hothouse tomato

Romaine and/or spinach leaves

Sea salt

Bragg Liquid Aminos

Assemble open-faced, spreading the avocado on bread, then the romaine and/or spinach leaves, then the tomato. Add a sprinkling of sea salt and a spritz of Bragg Liquid Aminos.

Power Rice & Rye

MENU ITEM #26/27

SERVES 6

2   cups brown rice

1   cup rye berries

3   cups water

3   cups vegetable broth

2   small carrots, chopped

1   celery stalk, chopped

1   cup finely chopped kale

½   onion, chopped

1   cup cut green beans

Bragg Liquid Aminos to taste

In a large saucepan, mix the brown rice, rye berries, 3 cups water, the vegetable broth, carrots, celery, kale, and onion. Bring to a boil over medium heat. Lower the heat, cover, and simmer 20 to 25 minutes, or until the rice and rye are tender and have absorbed the liquid. In a small saucepan, bring the green beans and ½ cup water to a boil. Cook 2 minutes and drain. Stir the green beens into the rice and rye and season with Bragg Liquid Aminos.

Steamed Veggies over Quinoa

MENU ITEM #28

SERVES 4

2 cups vegetable stock

1 cup quinoa, rinsed well

2 cups spinach

1 cup chopped broccoli

1 cup sliced zucchini

Bragg Liquid Aminos (or a pinch of sea salt and a bit of balsamic vinegar, if preferred)

In a small saucepan, bring the stock to a boil over medium heat, then add the quinoa. Stir to combine, return to a boil, then cover, reduce the heat to low, and cook 15 to 20 minutes, or until the liquid is absorbed. Fluff with a fork. Meanwhile, steam the vegetables using a steamer or a covered saucepan and a bit of water over low heat and season lightly with Bragg Liquid Aminos. To serve, mound the quinoa on a plate and cover with the vegetables.

Three-Grain Pilaf

MENU ITEM #29

SERVES 4

¼ cup hulled wheat berries

1 tablespoon olive oil

¼ cup wild rice

1½ cups water

¼ cup white wine

1 bay leaf

Salt and pepper to taste

¼ cup uncooked basmati rice

2 shallots, minced

1 cup (4 ounces weight) quartered shiitake mushrooms, stems removed

⅓ cup (2 ounces) chopped almonds with skins

4 green onions, thinly sliced

Soak the wheat berries 2 hours in enough water to cover, then drain. Put ½ tablespoon of the oil, the wheat berries, and the wild rice in a medium saucepan over medium heat and stir well. Add 1½ cups water, the wine, bay leaf, and salt and pepper to taste. Bring to a boil. Cover, lower the heat, and simmer 30 minutes. Stir in the basmati rice. Simmer, covered, 20 minutes more. Remove from the heat and allow to stand, covered. Heat the remaining ½ tablespoon oil in large skillet and sauté the shallots and shiitake mushrooms until softened, 3 to 4 minutes. Add the almonds and cook, stirring, 3 to 4 minutes. Stir in the green onions and cooked grains.

Angel Hair Pasta with Lemon and Garlic

MENU ITEM #30

SERVES 2

2 garlic cloves, chopped

2 tablespoons olive oil

2 cups white wine

2 tablespoons chopped fresh basil

1 fresh, firm tomato, chopped or diced

Juice of ½ lemon

½ pound whole-grain angel hair pasta

Freshly ground black pepper to taste

In a large sauté pan over medium-low heat, sauté the garlic in the olive oil just until it starts to brown. Add the wine and reduce by almost half. In the meantime, bring a large pot of water to a boil and cook the pasta until al dente, according to the package directions. When wine is reduced, remove it from the heat. Add the lemon juice, tomato, and basil and stir. Serve over the pasta and add freshly ground pepper to taste if you like.

Pasta Primavera

MENU ITEM #31

SERVES 4

1 ¼ cups vegetable stock

2 sprigs fresh thyme

Pinch of salt

½ cup diced carrots

1 cup broccoli florets

½ cup cauliflower florets

½ cup peas

1 pound whole-grain penne pasta

2 tablespoons olive oil

½ cup vegan parmesan (optional)

Bring a large pot of water to a boil. In a medium skillet, bring 1 cup of the stock to a boil. Add the thyme, salt, carrots, broccoli, and cauliflower and cook 6 to 7 minutes. Add the peas and cook until all the vegetables are tender. Turn off the heat. Salt the boiling water and cook the pasta according to the package directions. When the pasta is just about done, heat the vegetables again over medium heat, stirring in the olive oil and cooking about 1 minute. Add the remaining stock. Drain the pasta and toss with the vegetables. Top with the vegan parmesan.

Pasta with Fresh Vegetable Tomato Sauce

from Healthy Holidays

MENU ITEM #33

SERVES 6

- 1 tablespoon olive oil
- 2 small onions, diced
- 2 carrots, diced into ½-inch circles
- ¼ cup minced fresh parsley
  Salt and freshly ground black pepper
- 1 pound whole-grain pasta of your choice
- 2 28-ounce cans peeled or crushed tomatoes
- 2 small zucchini, cut in half lengthwise and sliced
- 1 ¼ cups vegetable broth
- ½ cup basil, cut into chiffonade
  tomatoes, undrained

In a large saucepan over medium-high heat, heat the oil. Add the onions and carrots, and sauté until lightly browned, about 5 to 7 minutes. Add the parsley and salt and pepper to taste. Stir in the tomatoes, including their juice, and the broth and simmer 10 minutes over low heat, breaking up the tomatoes with the back of a spoon. Add the zucchini and basil and cook another 5 minutes, or until the zucchini is tender. Bring a large pot of water to a boil over high heat and add 1 teaspoon salt. Drop in the pasta and cook until al dente, according to the package directions. Top the pasta with the sauce and serve.

Grilled Veggie Packets

MENU ITEM #35

SERVES 2

Place scrubbed red potatoes with skins, fresh green beans, sliced carrots, and sliced celery into aluminum foil packets (one per serving). Sprinkle with Bragg Liquid Aminos, olive oil, and garlic powder. Seal tight. Place by hot coals on the barbecue or in a 425°F oven for 40 minutes, or until done.

Baked Potato, Yam, or Sweet Potato
with Marinated Vegetables

MENU ITEM #37

SERVES 1

1 teaspoon mirin (Japanese sweet rice wine)

1 teaspoon rice vinegar

1 teaspoon Bragg Liquid Aminos

1 tablespoon sesame or olive oil

½ cucumber, peeled and then shaved into long strips with a peeler

½ carrot, peeled, cut in half lengthwise, and shaved into long strips with a peeler

½ large broccoli stem, peeled like a carrot and shaved into long strips with a peeler

1 medium potato, baked or cooked in the microwave, still steamy

In a medium bowl, whisk together the mirin, rice vinegar, Bragg Liquid Aminos, and oil. Add the vegetable strips and coat well. Set aside to marinate about 10 minutes. Cut open the potato and mash it with a fork. Spoon the vegetables over the potato and serve. If you have extra vegetables, use them to top mixed greens, and you have a matching salad!

Green Beans with Pine Nuts

from Healthy Life Kitchen

MENU ITEM #38
SERVES 6

2 pounds young green beans, ends trimmed
1 tablespoon salt
2 tablespoons soy margarine
1 tablespoon extra-virgin olive oil
⅓ cup pine nuts, lightly roasted

In a saucepan over high heat, bring enough water to cover the beans to a rolling boil. Add the beans and salt and lower the heat to medium-low. Cook until tender, about 6 to 7 minutes, and drain well. In a skillet over medium heat, melt the margarine with the oil. Add the beans and nuts to the pan, toss together, and serve at once.

Sautéed Broccoli Rabe

from Healthy Life Kitchen

MENU ITEM #39

SERVES 6

2   pounds broccoli rabe

1   tablespoon salt

1   tablespoon soy margarine

2   tablespoons extra-virgin olive oil

1   large garlic clove, cut into small pieces

Pinch of red pepper flakes

Using a sharp paring knife, peel the skin from the tough lower stalks of the broccoli rabe (most of the bottom portion of the stalk). Cut the broccoli rabe into roughly 3-inch lengths and rinse it well in a strainer. Fill a medium saucepan ¾ full of water and bring to a rolling boil over high heat. Add the broccoli rabe, cover partially, bring the water back to a boil, and cook 5 minutes, or until the broccoli rabe is crisp-tender. Meanwhile, place the salt, margarine, olive oil, garlic, and pepper flakes together in a cold skillet. Turn on the heat to low and sauté until the garlic starts to color, about 5 minutes. Do not let it brown.

Drain the broccoli rabe (but let some water cling to it) and transfer it to the skillet. Stir, cover, and cook gently, stirring occasionally until tender, about 5 minutes.

Eggless Salad

from Healthy Life Kitchen

MENU ITEM #42

SERVES 4

1 pound extra-firm tofu, drained thoroughly

1 teaspoon garlic powder

¼ to ½ cup Nayonaise, or to taste

1 teaspoon onion powder

1 to 2 tablespoons prepared organic mustard

Salt and pepper to taste

1 teaspoon cumin

1 medium carrot, chopped

Chopped scallions to taste (optional)

In a medium bowl, mash the tofu with a potato masher or fork. Add the Nayonaise, mustard, spices, and chopped vegetables, if desired. Refrigerate for at least 1 hour to allow flavors to mix. Serve on whole-grain bread.

Roasted Chicken with Garlic and Rosemary

from Healthy Life Kitchen

MENU ITEM #45

SERVES 4

  2 tablespoons soy margarine
  2 tablespoons olive oil
  2 garlic cloves
  1 free-range chicken, about 2½ pounds,
     cut into quarters
     Small sprig fresh rosemary
     Salt and freshly ground pepper
½ cup vermouth

Heat the soy margarine and oil in a large sauté pan over medium heat. When the margarine foams, add the garlic and the chicken quarters, skin side down. When the chicken is well browned on one side, turn the pieces over and add the rosemary.

When the chicken is cooked well on both sides, add a large pinch of salt and pepper and the vermouth. Allow the vermouth to bubble for about 3 minutes, then lower the heat to a simmer and cover the pan. Cook it for about 30 to 35 minutes, turning the chicken a couple of times. Transfer the chicken to a warm serving plate. Remove the garlic from the pan and discard. Tilt the pan and, with a spoon, remove and discard all but 2 tablespoons of fat. Return the pan to high heat, add 2 to 3 tablespoons water, and scrape up the cooking juices. Pour the juices over the chicken and serve.

Chinese-Style Steamed Fish

MENU ITEM #46

SERVES 2

Two 6-ounce cod fillets

Salt and freshly ground black pepper to taste

2 tablespoons dry vermouth

1 ½ teaspoons peeled, minced ginger

2 small garlic cloves, minced

4 teaspoons low-sodium tamari sauce

1 ½ teaspoons sesame oil

2 tablespoons chopped cilantro

Place a small cake rack in a large (12-inch-diameter) skillet and place a 9-inch-diameter glass pie dish on the rack. Put the fish in the dish and sprinkle lightly with salt and pepper. Sprinkle the vermouth, ginger, and garlic in the dish around the fish. Top the fish with the tamari sauce, sesame oil, and 1 tablespoon of the cilantro. Pour water into the skillet to a depth of 1 inch and bring the water to a boil over medium-low heat. Cover the skillet and steam the fish until just opaque in the center, about 10 minutes. Transfer the fish to plates. Top with the juices from the dish and the remaining cilantro.

Grilled Teriyaki Tofu or Fish

MENU ITEM #47

SERVES 1

 ½ cup tamari or low-sodium soy sauce

 3 tablespoons honey or Sucanat

 1 tablespoon mirin

 1 garlic clove, minced (or ½ teaspoon minced jarred garlic)

 ½ teaspoon dried ginger (or 1 teaspoon freshly grated ginger)

 2 extra-firm tofu steaks, cut into slices about ½-inch thick, or
    4 ounces fish of your choice

In a small saucepan over low heat, warm the marinade ingredients, stirring constantly until the flavors come together. Place the tofu or fish in a nonmetal bowl and pour the sauce on top. Marinate 20 minutes at room temperature (place in the refrigerator if marinating longer than 20 minutes). Grill 3 to 5 minutes on each side, or until the tofu is cooked through and the fish is flaky.

Spicy Grilled Salmon (or Chicken)

from Healthy Life Kitchen

MENU ITEM #48

SERVES 4

½ teaspoon salt

½ teaspoon cracked pepper

½ teaspoon garlic powder

¼ teaspoon cayenne pepper

¼ teaspoon paprika

4 salmon fillets or 4 boneless,
   skinless chicken breasts

½ teaspoon olive oil

Mix all the dry seasonings together. Rub the salmon or chicken with olive oil and then coat with the dry seasonings. Grill over a very hot grill for 3 to 5 minutes on each side for fish, 7 to 10 minutes on each side for chicken.

Herb-Infused Whole Baked Fish

from Healthy Life Kitchen

MENU ITEM #49

SERVES 4

2 tablespoons olive oil

1 large yellow onion, chopped

1 whole fish (striped bass, red snapper, or trout works well), cleaned

1 bunch rosemary

1 bunch marjoram

½ cup white wine

Olive oil or spray

1 garlic clove, minced

1 bunch parsley

Preheat the oven to 400°F. In a sauté pan over medium-low heat, heat the olive oil. Add the onion and cook until golden brown, about 5 minutes. Stuff the fish with half the marjoram, half the rosemary, and half the onion. Place the fish in an oil-sprayed baking dish. Add the white wine and garlic to the onion remaining in the pan and sauté over low heat for about 7 minutes, or until the alcohol is burned off. Pour this mixture over the fish and surround the fish with the remaining marjoram and rosemary and the parsley. Bake the fish for 10 minutes per each inch of thickness.

Classic Bruschetta

from Healthy Life Kitchen

MENU ITEM #50
SERVES 4 TO 6

8 plum tomatoes, chopped and seeded

8 basil leaves, chopped

1 or 2 garlic cloves, minced

2 teaspoons olive oil

   Salt and freshly ground black pepper to taste

1 French baguette, sliced thin and toasted

In a small bowl, combine the tomatoes, basil, garlic, olive oil, salt, and pepper. Spoon the mixture on top of the toasted bread and serve immediately.

Sweet Pea Guacamole

MENU ITEM #55

SERVES 6

1-pound bag frozen peas
½ large avocado
1 teaspoon fresh lime juice
¼ cup fresh cilantro leaves, chopped (optional)
Salt and freshly ground black pepper to taste

Place the peas in a medium saucepan and fill the pan halfway up with water. Bring to a boil over high heat and cook 3 to 5 minutes, or until the peas are soft. Drain and set aside. Cut the avocado into chunks. In a food processor, add the cooked peas and mix until smooth. Add the avocado chunks and continue to process until smooth. Add the lime juice, cilantro, salt, and pepper, and process a few more seconds until smooth. Chill, covered, for 1 to 2 hours and serve with baked tortilla chips.

Fresh Fruit Sorbet

MENU ITEM #59

SERVES 4

4 cups seedless red grapes (1 to 1½ pounds), washed

1 cup 100 percent pomegranate (or other favorite) juice

2 tablespoons fresh lime juice

⅛ cup Sucanat

Fresh mint for garnish

Place the grapes in a 13-×-9-inch baking pan and freeze. Transfer to a food processor. Add the juice, lime, and Sucanat and pulse until fairly smooth. Put back into the pan and freeze 1 hour. Stir, then freeze 30 minutes, or until the desired consistency. Scoop into glasses and add the mint garnish.

I had the opportunity to coach in Booty School, and loved the concept of eating mini-meals and having a contract. It was the type of structure many of us need when learning new things.

—DAR,
Marilu.com
member

Appendix

Marilu Henner's Food-Combining Chart

CHART ONE

DO NOT COMBINE FOODS FROM CHARTS ONE AND TWO

← DO NOT → COMBINE

STARCHES

Potatoes •
Carrots • Parsnips •
Corn • Winter Squash •
Grains (barley, buckwheat,
dried corn, oats, rice,
wheat, rye) • Pasta •
Bread • Brown Rice •
Wild Rice

LEGUMES

**(May be combined
with grains, pasta,
bread to make
complete protein)**

Beans • Peas •
Tofu • Peanuts

PROTEINS

Meats* • Poultry •
Fish • Cheese, Milk,
and Other Dairy
Products* • Eggs •
Nuts** • Seeds

*I don't recommend eating dairy
or meats. However, I've included
these for those who choose
to eat these foods.
**Nuts have so much fat
that they should always
be eaten with an acid fruit

OK TO COMBINE

VEGETABLES

Cabbage • Kale • Lettuce •
Celery • Sprouts • Artichokes •
Mushrooms • String Beans •
Green Peas • Green Beans •
Red, Yellow, and Green Peppers •
Cucumber • Cauliflower •
Broccoli • Spinach • Tomatoes

OK TO COMBINE

OILS AND FATS

Butter • Margarine •
All Oils (including olive,
vegetable and safflower) •
Avocados • Olives • Coconuts

Marilu Henner's Food-Combining Chart

CHART TWO

DO NOT COMBINE FOODS FROM CHARTS ONE AND TWO

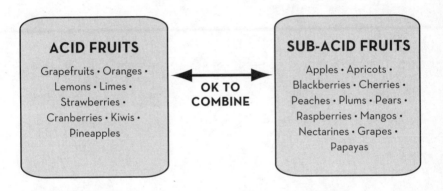

ACID FRUITS

Grapefruits • Oranges •
Lemons • Limes •
Strawberries •
Cranberries • Kiwis •
Pineapples

OK TO COMBINE

SUB-ACID FRUITS

Apples • Apricots •
Blackberries • Cherries •
Peaches • Plums • Pears •
Raspberries • Mangos •
Nectarines • Grapes •
Papayas

SWEET FRUITS

DO NOT COMBINE WITH OTHER FOODS

Bananas • Plantains • Dates •
Persimmons • Figs • Prunes •
Raisins • Dried Fruits

MELONS

DO NOT COMBINE WITH OTHER FOODS

Cantaloupe • Honeydew •
Watermelon • Casaba •
Christmas • Crenshaw

Acknowledgments

It's never easy writing a book. It's a lot like having a baby—only harder! But from the beginning, this book was truly a labor of love because of the following people:

To Cassie Jones, editor extraordinaire. I can't believe it's our fifth book together, and it only gets better. Thank you for your patience, insight, and expertise. You are the BEST!

To her team at HarperCollins: Ruth Mannes, Johnathan Wilber, Diane Aronson, Helen Song, Richard Ljoenes, Lorie Pagnozzi, and Jessica Peskay. To Steve Ross and Margot Schupf for this wonderful opportunity. To Mary Ellen O'Neill, who with Cassie Jones visited Marilu.com, saw what we do there, and decided to have me share it with the rest of the world through this book. Thank you for your support and patience, and for welcoming me into the Collins family. To Patrick McCarthy, Karen Kleber, and Bill Westmoreland—shooting a cover has never been so easy. A big thank-you to Jean Marie Kelly, and, of course, to Paul Olsewski, who knows how to promote a life better than anyone. Our seventh book together, and we never run out of good times and stories. Thank you.

To the one and only Donald Trump, his impressive children, Ivanka and Donald, Jr., and my stellar *Celebrity Apprentice* teammates: Trace Adkins, Carol Alt, Stephen Baldwin, Nadia Comaneci, Tiffany Fallon, Jennie Finch, Nely Galán, Lennox Lewis, Piers Morgan, Omarosa, Tito Ortiz, Vinnie Pastore, and Gene Simmons. We are bonded forever. Thanks for the great time (and extra material) that only made this book better.

Once again I had the best life team roster working behind the scenes, including the incomparable Richard Feldstein and Dennis Romero at Nigro, Karlin, Segal, & Feldstein; the fearless Dick Guttman and the no-nonsense Susan Madore of Guttman and Associates; my talented agent, Jonathan Howard of Innovative Artists; and my dynamic manager, Rory Rosegarten of The Conversation Company. I also had my fabulous Web site team at Marilu.com and our online classes, which were the heartbeat of this book. My undying gratitude to Tonia Kulberda, without whom nothing is possible; Mary Beth Borkowski, the guardian angel of Marilu.com; and all the coaches and members, including Cathy Dodd, Reiko Dyer, Rosemary Guidry, Laure Lovelace, Carol Melnick, Jill Nelson, Doris Pendergrass, Cindy Raschke, and Faith Waite who all contributed to the message of this book.

To Robert Lieberman, who shares with me the two best members of any team, Nick and Joey. And to the rest of my extraordinary book team: Thank you, MaryAnn Hennings and Elizabeth Carney, for their continued support and culinary expertise; Kaisha Trzaska, for being a naturally gifted writer and a beacon of insight, and for keeping the book team in line with your steady, calming influence; Ella Dwyer, who was so good at mining the gold from the Marilu.com chats and for being my very own apprentice; Monika Music, for your organization skills, cheery attitude, and helping me with the kids; to my rambitious (his word) son Joey, whose speed on the keyboard is almost as fast as his speed on the gridiron; and to my clever son Nick—a future author in his own right—whose presence joyfully reminded me how determined I was to have a child years ago while writing my first book. Here I was, proudly working side-by-side with him fourteen years later on my eighth. To my brother, coauthor, and partner in crime, Lorin Henner: As usual, there are no words to describe how great it is to work with you. To be able to do what I love with someone I love so much is a true gift. Your talent, intelligence, focus, and unparalleled sense of humor (not to mention ability to cat-nap) made it easy to work this hard with someone so much fun!

And to my darling, handsome husband, Michael, who first came into my life when we were college kids and found me again when we were both ready. Thank you for understanding how crazy it is around here when the whole house is in Book Hell. I couldn't love anyone more than I love you.

With all these wonderful people, no wonder I get to wear my life well!

Index

acetaldehyde, 59
acetate, 59
acting, as process of transformation, 104–106
acting exercises
    character development, 123–126
    finding self within self, 108–110
    finding your objective, 126–127
    food for thought, 115–117
    for healthy living, 106–108
    observation, 110–114
    playing new "you," 130–133
    props and costumes, 127–130
    The Rant, 117–119
    sense memory, 120–122
aging process
    brain and, 153–154
    healthy living and, 49–51, 73–79, 179–180
    use it or lose it principle and, 151–152
alcohol, 58, 59–60, 74, 183
Alderman, Tom, 166–167, 168

alignment technique, 168
angel hair pasta with lemon and garlic, 232
anger, 30–31, 118
appearance, 172–176
apple-shaped women, 65
arsenic, 74
attitude
    importance of, 10
    negative, 143–144, 181, 182
    positive, 10–11, 143–144, 181, 182
authority, questioning, 189–191
automobiles, 100–101
avocado, lettuce, and tomato (ALT) sandwich, 228

balance, 35
bathroom cabinets, 95
bathroom organization, 94–96
bedrooms, 98–99
beets, 221, 222
Bergman, Sandahl, 170
black tea, 74

B-L-A-S-T (Bored, Lonely, Angry, Starving, or Tired), 42
blood pressure, 64
body armor, 31–34
body issues
    mother-daughter relationship and, 36
    sexuality and, 195, 196
body language, 108, 139, 167
body mass index (BMI), 64, 65
body shape, 65, 175–176
Booty Camp Blitz
    5-day contract, 204–206
    menus, 207–212
    recipes, 213–247
boredom, 42
brain
    exercise, 153–154
    sex and, 193–197
breast cancer, 60
broccoli rabe, sautéed, 238
Brooks, Jim, xi–xii
Brown, Michael, 66–70
bruschetta, 245

caffeine, 55
cancer, 51, 60, 63, 65, 71–72
Carlisle, Kitty, 18
cars, 100–101
Celebrity Apprentice, xiv–xv, 4–8, 138
centered foods, 58
change
    failure to sustain, 104
    fear of, 14–15
    stress of, 179–180
character creation, 128–130
character development exercise, 123–126
chicken with garlic and rosemary, roasted, 240

childhood
    feelings about, 21
    food patterns learned in, 29
    lack of skills learned in, 35
    sexual impressions from, 196
Chinese medicine, 76
chlorine, 74
cholesterol, 64–65
chronic disease, 51
closet organization, 96–98
clothing, 96–98
clothing style, 174–176
coffee, 74
colon, 75
colon therapy, 75
comfort zones
    analyzing your, 3
    challenging your, 4–6
    increased responsibilities and, 2
    personal, 2–8
communication
    listening skills, 139–143
    nonverbal, 139
    presentation and, 166–167
    resilience and, 146–148
    skills, 163–166
    in work situations, 167–168
concentrated foods, 56–57
control, self-sabotage and, 40–41
conversational rhythms, 140–141
cravings, 43, 54
Crystal, Billy, 145

daikon soup, 215
dairy products, 53–54, 55–56
daughters, mothers and, 36
death, fear of, 16–17
deep-tissue massage, 78
dehydration, 74–75
dental health, 76–77

depression, 118
destructive behavior. *See*
    self-sabotage
detox process
    benefits of, 73–75
    healing crisis from, 54–56
    suggestions for, 75–79
diabetes, 65
diet. *See also* eating; food
    effects of, on health, 60–64
    normal, 71–73
diets, fad, 50–51
disease
    body shape and, 65
    diet and, 63–64
    fear of, 16–17
doctors, 60–64, 66
dressings, 216–217

eating. *See also* food; overeating
    changing habits of, 50–82
    emotional, 28–29, 42
    feelings about, 30
    out of boredom, 42
eating exercise, 115–117
eggless salad, 239
emotional eating, 28–29, 42
emotions. *See* feelings
environment, organizing for health,
    85–101
environmental toxins, 74
exercise
    benefits of, 155–157
    brain, 153–154
    for detox, 77–78
    finding enjoyable, 158
    health and, 63, 64
    importance of regular, 154–155
    mini-workouts, 205
    as stress reliever, 183

tips for, 158–162
    variety in, 6
exercise clothing, 159
exfoliation, 78–79
expectations, 181–182
eye contact, 167
eyes, 139

"Face Your Fears" questionnaire, 11–12
fad diets, 50–51
failure
    fear of, 17–18
    resilience after, 146–148
familiarity, 180
family relationships, 124–125,
    186–188
fat distribution, 65
fathers, sons and, 36. *See also* parents
fatty foods, 52
fear
    of change, 14–15
    of death/illness, 16–17
    deep-rooted, 187–188
    embracing your, 9–11
    of failure, 17–18
    of imperfection, 15–16
    of losing weight, 13–14
    of success, 14, 40
    of unknown, 180
feedback, 143–144
feelings
    negative, 22–23
    understanding your, 20–21,
        121–122
    venting, 117–119
fish
    baked, 244
    Chinese-style steamed, 241
    grilled salmon, 243
    grilled teriyaki, 242

food. *See also* eating
    centered, 58
    concentrated, 56–57
    cravings, 43, 54
    eliminating health robbing,
        53–56
    fatty, 52
    healthy, 51–53
    junk, 52, 90
    as preventive medicine, 62–64
    processed, 53, 55
    raw, 54
    seduction of, 30
    self-sabotage and, 25–26
    wet, 56–57
food addictions, overcoming, 52–53
food-combining chart, 249–250
food comfort zone, challenging your,
    5–6
food industry, 72–73
forgiveness, for self, 18
Forrest, Frederic, 67, 128–129
Fosse, Bob, 169, 170–171
fruits, 53
fruit sorbet, 247

garage organization, 99–100
goals, 126–127
grains, 231
green beans with pine nuts, 237
guacamole, sweet pea, 246
gym
    exercise at, 155
    self-consciousness at, 9–10

Hagen, Uta, 127–128
hair style, 173
headaches, from detox process, 55
health
    advice, 60–61
    role of diet and exercise in, 44,
        60–64
health industry, growth of, 50–51
healthy food, 51–53
healthy living
    aging process and, 49–51, 73–79
    principles of, 60–61
    transforming self for, 103–108
heart disease, 65
Hippocrates, 64
hobbies, 183
home environment
    bathrooms, 94–96
    bedrooms, 98–99
    closets, 96–98
    garage, 99–100
    kitchens, 88–94
    morning routine and, 85–87
    organizing for health, 85–101
human growth hormone (HGH),
    53
hunger, 28–29
hypertension, 63

ideal life, imagining your, 1–2
illness, fear of, 16–17
imagination, lack of, 42
immune system, 71–72, 152
imperfection, fear of, 15–16
information
    fear of too much, 16–17
    questioning validity of, 189–191
infrared saunas, 78
interpersonal communication. *See*
    communication

jealousy, 34–36
job interviews, 167–168
job stress, 186
junk food, 52, 53, 90

kitchen organization, 88–94

lead, 74
L-Glutamine, 59
Lieberman, Robert, 67
life design, 1–2
listening skills, 139–143
liver damage, from alcohol
    consumption, 59
liver detox, 75, 76
lymphatic system, 76

macrobiotics, 58
makeup areas, 95–96
makeup style, 173–174
mannerisms, 107–108
Martin, Ed Kaye, 118, 119
meal preparation, kitchen
    organization and, 90–92
medical school curriculum, 63
medication, 63
meditation, 184
memory loss, 153
menstrual cycle, 36–37
mercury, 74
mercury fillings, 77
messiness, 185
milk, 74
minerals, 74–75
mini-workouts, 205
misinformation, 189–191
misplaced anger, 30–31
money stress, 185–186
morning routine, 85–88
mothers, daughters and, 36. See also
    parents
muscle memory, 106, 108

negative attitude, 143–144, 181, 182
negative feelings, 22–23

nonverbal communication, 139
nori salad wrap, 226
normal diet, 71–73

obesity, 51, 65
objective, defining your, 126–127
observation exercise, 110–114
opportunities, missed, 125–126
oral hygiene, 76–77
organization
    bathroom, 94–96
    closet, 96–98
    garage, 99–100
    kitchen, 88–94
    morning routine and, 85–88
    need for, 83–85
    rules for, 93
osteoporosis, 160
overeating
    bloated feeling from, 37
    emotional eating and, 28–29
    negative feelings and, 22
    self-sabotage and, 30–32
    stopping, 43
    triggers for, 42
overweight
    avoiding sexuality and, 33–34
    as body armor, 31–32
    stress due to, 186

parents
    early imprinting from, 196
    father-son relationships, 36
    feelings toward, 21, 35
    mother-daughter relationships, 36
    overindulgent, 181–182
party personalities, 136–138
pasta
    angel hair, with lemon and garlic,
        232

pasta (*continued*)
    with fresh vegetable tomato
        sauce, 234
    pasta primavera, 233
perception, 193–194
perfectionism, 15–16
personal interactions
    listening skills for, 139–143
    personality and, 135–136
personality development, 135–136
personality types, 136–138
personal style, 172–176
pharmaceutical industry, 63,
    190–191
physical inactivity, 154–155
Pilates, 157
plan B situations, 144–146
positive attitude, 10–11, 143–144,
    181, 182
posture, 108, 111
potatoes, baked, 236
potato-shaped men, 65
premenstrual syndrome (PMS),
    36–37
preparation, 169–171
presentation
    communication skills and,
        163–166
    importance of, 163, 166–167
    personal style and, 172–176
present moment, staying in,
    164–166
President's Fitness Challenge, 158
preventive medicine, 62–64, 64–66
private moments, 111–112
processed foods, 53, 55
Project Runway, 8
public speaking, 166–167

quinoa, 230

rant exercise, 117–119
raw foods, 54
rebounding, 78
recipes, 213–247
red meat, 53, 56
reflexology, 76
relationships
    family, 124–125, 186–188
    parental, 21, 35–36
    sexuality and, 197–201
    stressful, 188–189
resilience, 146–148
rice
    power rice and rye, 229
    three-grain pilaf, 231
rock bottom, 22–23

salad dressings, 216–217
salads
    eggless, 239
    grilled vegetable S, 219
    Japanese baby greens, 220
    nori salad wrap, 226
    salade Niçoise, 223
    salad with beets, 221
    taco salad, 224
    tuna and asparagus, 225
    warm veggie, 218
salmon, spicy grilled, 243
sandwiches
    avocado, lettuce, and tomato
        (ALT), 228
    tomato and basil, 227
saunas, 78
Savant, Doug, 131
seeds, 54
self, forgiveness of, 18
self-analysis, 116–117
self-consciousness
    about appearance, 41

in acting, 143–144
at the gym, 9–10
perception and, 141–142
sexuality and, 195, 197–198
in social situations, 142–143, 148
self-criticism, 10–11
self-depreciation, 183
self-image, sexuality and, 33–34
self-observation, 107–110
self-sabotage
    avoiding sexuality, 33–34
    body armor and, 31–32
    control and, 40–41
    emotional eating, 28–29, 42
    fear of success and, 40
    food and, 25–26, 30
    jealousy and, 34–36
    misplaced anger, 30–31
    PMS and, 36–37
    reasons for, 28, 38–40
    resolving, 42–46
    through lack of imagination, 42
    understanding, 25–27
self-transformation, for healthy
    living, 103–108
self-within exercise, 108–110
sense memories, 120–122
sex
    brain and, 193–197
    mindset for, 197–198, 199–201
    pleasure principle, 198–201
    use it or lose it principle and, 152
sexual fantasies, 195, 198, 199–200
sexuality
    avoiding, 33–34
    influences on, 196–197
    self-consciousness and, 195, 197–198
Sharon, Ruth Velikovsky, 20, 34
situations, ability to read, 139–143
skepticism, 189–191

skin brushing, 78–79
sleep routine, 86–88
smiling, 168
snooze alarms, 86–87
social interactions, need for regular,
    154
social situations
    ability to read others in, 139–143
    handling unexpected, 144–146
    self-consciousness in, 142–143, 148
soft drinks, 74
sons, fathers and, 36
soups
    creamy daikon, 215
    Joey's "chicken" soup, 214
    spinach, 213
spinach soup, 213
spontaneity, 145
sprouts, 54
Stone, Sharon, 165
strength-training exercises, 160
stress
    attitude and, 181–182
    change and, 179–180
    coping with, 183–184
    increased responsibilities and, 2
    sources of, 184–189
stress relievers, 183–184
style, 172–176
submissiveness, 31
success
    attitude for, 182–183
    fear of, 14, 40
sugar, 53, 55
sweet pea guacamole, 246
sweet potatoes, baked, 236

taco salad, 224
talk shows, 164–165
tap water, 75

teeth, 76–77
therapists, qualities of good, 18–19
therapy, 18–21, 113–114
tofu
    eggless salad, 239
    grilled teriyaki, 242
tomato and basil sandwich, 227
Total Health Makeover (THM)
    program, 13
toxins, 74
traffic, 184–185
tuna and asparagus salad, 225

unexpected situations, 144–146
unhealthy foods, eliminating, 53–56
use it or lose it principle, 151–152

vegetables, 53, 55, 236
    balsamic marinated beets, 222
    green beans with pine nuts, 237

grilled veggie packs, 235
    marinated, 236
    sautéed broccoli rabe, 238
    steamed, over quinoa, 230
vegetable salads, 218–221
vegetable soup, 214

waistline measurements, 65
water, 57, 74–75
weight loss
    backsliding and, 38–40
    elimination of dairy and,
        55–56
    fear of, 13–14
    misplaced anger and, 30–31
    sexuality and, 33–34
weight stress, 186
wet foods, 56–57

yams, baked, 236